Certified Coding Associate (CCA) Exam Preparation

Ninth Edition

Rachael Gagner D'Andrea
MS, RHIA, CDIP, CHTS-TR, CPHQ

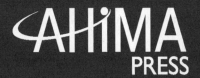

AHIMA PRESS

ISBN: 978-1-58426-863-5
eISBN: 978-1-58426-864-2

AHIMA Product No.: AC400321

AHIMA Staff:
Jessica Block, MA, Production Development Editor
Sarah Cybulski, MA, Assistant Editor
Megan Grennan, Director, Content Production and AHIMA Press
James Pinnick, Vice President, Content and Learning Solutions
Christine Scheid, Content Development Manager
Rachel Schratz, MA, Associate Digital Content Developer

Cover image: © 31moonlight31; iStock

For more information, including updates, about AHIMA Press publications, visit http://www.ahima.org /education/press.

American Health Information Management Association
233 North Michigan Avenue, 21st Floor
Chicago, Illinois 60601-5809
ahima.org

Contents

About the Contributing Editor

Rachael Gagner D'Andrea, MS, RHIA, CDIP, CHTS-TR, CPHQ, is a consultant and instructor for the State of Connecticut and lecturer for the State of Florida college systems. She is past president of the Connecticut Health Information Management Association (CtHIMA) and an editor and technical reviewer for multiple publications.

With over 30 years of experience in health information management (HIM), her career has encompassed several domains, including acute care, quality improvement, home health, software marketing and development, and education. She is a past director for CtHIMA, previous member of AHIMA's Clinical Practice Council, and contributor to the Agency for Healthcare Research and Quality's ICD-10-CM/PCS transition workgroup. She has lectured extensively on coding, diagnosis-related groups, reimbursement, and data quality issues throughout the United States and internationally.

As an educator—both nationally and internationally—and an active committee member of AHIMA's Assembly on Education, Envision, National Association for Healthcare Quality, and as an ICD-10 expert, Ms. D'Andrea continues to advance her knowledge in our dynamic profession with the observation that we in HIM are never finished learning. She promotes and supports this direction for all HIM professionals.

Ms. D'Andrea has her master's degree in health informatics and information management from the College of St. Scholastica.

Acknowledgments

AHIMA Press would like to thank Dianna Foley, RHIA, CCS, CDIP, CHPS, Gretchen Jopp, MS, RHIA, CCS, CPC, and Cari Greenwood, RHIA, CCS, CICA, CPC, for serving as technical reviewers of this edition.

Additionally, AHIMA Press would like to thank Gretchen Jopp for authoring new items for the instructor-only exam that accompanies this book.

About the CCA Exam

Coding professionals who hold the CCA credential have demonstrated coding competency across all settings, including hospitals and physician practices.

Since 2002, the CCA designation has been a nationally recognized standard of achievement in the health information management (HIM) field.

CCAs:

- Exhibit a level of commitment, competency, and professional capability that is valued by employers.
- Demonstrate a commitment to the coding profession.
- Distinguish themselves from others as having passed AHIMA's rigorous CCA exam.

For exam eligibility requirements and more, visit AHIMA's Certification website at https://www.ahima.org/certification-careers/certification-exams/cca/.

CCA Exam Domains and Tasks

Domain 1: Clinical Classification Systems

Tasks:

1. Interpret healthcare data for code assignment
2. Incorporate clinical vocabularies and terminologies used in health information systems
3. Abstract pertinent information from medical records
4. Consult reference materials to facilitate code assignment
5. Apply inpatient coding guidelines
6. Apply outpatient coding guidelines
7. Apply physician coding guidelines
8. Assign inpatient codes
9. Assign outpatient codes
10. Assign physician codes
11. Sequence codes according to healthcare setting
12. Determine an Evaluation and Management (E/M) Level (history, exam, medical decision making, or time)
13. Use of appropriate modifiers

Domain 2: Reimbursement Methodologies

Tasks:

1. Sequence codes for appropriate reimbursement
2. Link diagnoses and CPT® codes according to payer specific guidelines
3. Understand DRG methodology
4. Understand APC methodology
5. Evaluate NCCI edits
6. Reconcile NCCI edits
7. Validate medical necessity using LCD and NCD
8. Understand claim form types
9. Communicate with financial departments

10. Evaluate claim denials
11. Process claim denials
12. Communicate with the physician to clarify documentation
13. Knowledge of Hierarchical Condition Categories (HCC) and risk adjustment
14. Application of CPT guidelines around bundling and unbundling

Domain 3: Health Records and Data Content

Tasks:

1. Retrieve medical record
2. Analyze medical records quantitatively for completeness
3. Analyze medical records qualitatively for deficiencies
4. Perform data abstraction
5. Request patient-specific documentation from other sources (ancillary depts., physician's office, etc.)
6. Retrieve patient information from master patient index
7. Educate providers on health data standards
8. Interpret coding data reports
9. Understand the different components of the medical record

Domain 4: Compliance

Tasks:

1. Identify discrepancies between coded data and supporting documentation
2. Validate that codes assigned by provider or electronic systems are supported by proper documentation
3. Perform ethical coding
4. Clarify documentation through ethical physician query
5. Research latest coding changes for fee/charge ticket and chargemaster
6. Implement latest coding changes for fee/charge ticket and chargemaster
7. Educate providers on compliant coding
8. Assist in preparing the organization for external audits

Domain 5: Information Technologies

Tasks:

1. Navigate throughout the EHR
2. Utilize encoding and grouping software
3. Utilize practice management and HIM systems
4. Utilize CAC software that automatically assigns codes based on electronic text
5. Validate the codes assigned by CAC software

Domain 6: Confidentiality and Privacy

Tasks:

1. Ensure patient confidentiality (HIPAA, state regulations, etc.)
2. Educate healthcare staff on privacy and confidentiality issues

3. Recognize and report privacy issues/violations
4. Maintain a secure work environment
5. Utilize passcodes/passwords
6. Access only minimal necessary documents/information
7. Release patient-specific data to authorized individuals
8. Protect electronic documents/protected health information (PHI) through encryption
9. Transfer electronic documents through secure sites
10. Retain confidential records appropriately
11. Destroy confidential records appropriately
12. Understand information blocking

How to Use This Book and Online Assessment

The CCA practice questions and practice exams in this book and on the accompanying website test knowledge of content pertaining to the CCA competencies published by AHIMA and available at https://www.ahima.org/certification-careers/certification-exams/cca/. The multiple-choice practice questions and exams in this book and the accompanying website are presented in a similar format to those that might be found on the CCA examination.

This book contains 200 multiple choice practice questions and two multiple choice practice exams (with 100 questions each). Because each question is aligned to one of the six CCA domains, you will be able to determine whether you need knowledge or skill building in particular areas of the exam domains. Each question provides an answer rationale and reference with the correct answer. Pursuing the sources of these references will help you build your knowledge and skills in specific domains.

To most effectively use this book, work through all of the practice questions first. This will help you identify areas in which you may need further preparation. For the questions that you answer incorrectly, read the associated references to help refresh your knowledge. After going through the practice questions, take one of the practice exams. Again, for the questions that you answer incorrectly, refresh your knowledge by reading the associated references. Continue in the same manner with the second practice exam.

Retake the practice questions and exams as many times as you like. Remember that to help build your knowledge and skills, you should review the references provided for all questions that you answered incorrectly.

The website presents the same CCA practice questions and two-timed practice exams printed in the book. These exams can be run in practice mode, which allows you to work at your own pace, or exam mode, which simulates the timed exam experience. The practice questions and simulated practice exams can be set to be presented in random order, or you may choose to go through the questions in sequential order by domain. You may also choose to practice or test your skills on specific domains. For example, if you would like to build your skills in domain 2, you may choose only domain 2 questions for a given practice session.

Test-Taking Tips

The best way to prepare for the CCA certification exam is to study the material you have learned over the course of your health information management educational program. Because it is difficult to remember everything you have learned over the course of the program, it is important to review the information. This is best done using this exam preparation guide and the tips found in the How to Use This Book and Online Assessment section. Carefully review the information about the CCA exam found at https://www.ahima.org/certification-careers/certification-exams/cca/. You will want to prepare yourself mentally, physically, and emotionally to succeed.

Other tips for studying:
- Be sure to get enough sleep.
- Eat a healthy, well-balanced diet.
- Stay hydrated.
- Take breaks.
- Get some exercise.
- Do not try to memorize everything; work at understanding.
- Use tricks to remember the material, like using an acronym or other type of word or visual association.
- Try to eliminate other stressors, if possible.
- Take a practice exam in the two-hour time frame you will have for the exam.
- If you do not know where the testing center is located, visit it before the day of the exam. This will help you avoid getting lost or being late for your exam.

Exam Day Tips

- Get enough sleep in the days leading up to the exam.
- Wear comfortable clothes and dress in layers so that you can remove or add a layer based on the temperature of the room.
- Eat a healthy breakfast and give yourself enough time to get ready to leave so you are not rushed.
- Arrive at the testing center 30 minutes prior to your exam time with your required identification.
- You will have two hours to complete the exam. Do not obsess over the clock in the room, but do budget your time. This should allow you to answer each question and review any questions you may want to revisit. Time management will be an important part of taking the exam.
- Be sure to read each question carefully. Do not automatically assume you know the answer to a question without first reading the entire question and each answer choice carefully. After reviewing each answer, choose the best answer.
- Skip questions that you do not know the answer to or that are difficult and come back to them. You may find something in another question that helps you to recall information you need to answer a question you skipped. Be sure to manage your time well while you do this.
- Be sure to answer every test question. A guess is better than not taking the opportunity to answer a question. But do so after carefully reviewing the question and the possible answers. After eliminating answers you know are incorrect, make the best selection. A true guess will give you a one-in-four chance of getting a question correct.
- Remember to relax as much as possible and BREATHE. You can do this!

PRACTICE QUESTIONS

Domain 1 | *Clinical Classification Systems*

1. Identify the diagnosis code for carcinoma in situ of vocal cord.

   a. D02.0

   b. C32.0

   c. D49.1

   d. D14.1

2. Identify the diagnosis code(s) for melanoma of skin of right shoulder.

   a. D03.61, C43.61

   b. C43.61

   c. C43.60

   d. D03.61

3. Which of the following organizations is responsible for updating the procedure classification of ICD-10-PCS?

   a. Centers for Disease Control (CDC)

   b. Centers for Medicare and Medicaid Services (CMS)

   c. National Center for Health Statistics (NCHS)

   d. World Health Organization (WHO)

4. In ICD-10-CM, a condition that is produced by another illness or an injury and remains after the acute phase of the illness or injury is referred to as a:

   a. Late effect

   b. Sequela

   c. Complication

   d. Comorbidity

5. Which character in an ICD-10-CM diagnosis code provides information regarding encounter of care?

   a. Fourth

   b. Fifth

   c. Sixth

   d. Seventh

6. What does the fourth character of an ICD-10-CM diagnosis code capture?

   a. Anatomic site

   b. Severity

   c. Etiology

   d. Supplemental information

7. ICD-10-CM codes must be a minimum length of how many characters?

    a. Three

    b. Five

    c. Six

    d. Seven

8. Notes appearing under a three-character code apply to which of the following?

    a. Only to category codes that are exactly three-characters long

    b. To all codes within that category

    c. Only to one specific code

    d. To all codes within that chapter

9. Which volume of ICD-10-CM contains the Tabular and Alphabetic Index of procedures?

    a. Volume 1

    b. Volume 2

    c. Volume 3

    d. None of the above

10. An exception to the Excludes 1 definition is the circumstance when the two conditions _____.

    a. Are unrelated to each other

    b. Are related to each other

    c. Will not be assigned as the principal diagnosis

    d. Are injuries with external cause codes

11. Identify the correct diagnosis code(s) for adenoma of left adrenal cortex with Conn's syndrome.

    a. D35.02, E26.01

    b. D35.02

    c. E26.01

    d. E26.01, D35.7

12. Which of the following is a standard terminology used to code medical procedures and services?

    a. CPT

    b. HCPCS

    c. ICD-10-PCS

    d. SNOMED CT

13. Identify the appropriate ICD-10-CM diagnosis code for right cerebral contusion with 15-minute loss of consciousness, initial encounter for care.

    a. T14.8

    b. S06.371A

    c. S06.311A

    d. S06.310A

14. If a patient has an excision of a malignant lesion of the skin, the CPT code is determined by the body area from which the excision occurs and which of the following?

    a. Length of the lesion as described in the pathology report

    b. Dimension of the specimen submitted as described in the pathology report

    c. Width times the length of the lesion as described in the operative report

    d. Diameter of the lesion as well as the most narrow margins required to adequately excise the lesion described in the operative report

15. According to CPT, a repair of a laceration that includes retention sutures would be considered what type of closure?

    a. Simple

    b. Intermediate

    c. Complex

    d. Not specified

16. A patient is admitted with spotting. She had been treated two weeks previously for a miscarriage with sepsis. The sepsis had resolved, and she is afebrile at this time. She is treated with an aspiration dilation and curettage and products of conception are found. Which of the following should be the principal diagnosis?

    a. Miscarriage

    b. Complications of spontaneous abortion with sepsis

    c. Sepsis

    d. Spontaneous abortion with sepsis

17. An 80-year-old female is admitted with fever, lethargy, hypotension, tachycardia, oliguria, and elevated WBC. The patient has more than 100,000 organisms of *Escherichia coli* per cc of urine. The attending physician documents "urosepsis." How should the coding professional proceed to code this case?

    a. Code sepsis as the principal diagnosis with urinary tract infection due to *E. coli* as secondary diagnosis.

    b. Code urinary tract infection with sepsis as the principal diagnosis.

    c. Query the physician to determine if the patient has sepsis due to the symptomatology.

    d. Query the physician to determine if the patient has septic shock so that this may be used as the principal diagnosis.

18. A 65-year-old patient, with a history of lung cancer, is admitted to a healthcare facility with ataxia and syncope and a fractured arm as a result of falling. The patient undergoes a closed reduction of the fracture in the emergency department and undergoes a complete workup for metastatic carcinoma of the brain. The patient is found to have metastatic carcinoma of the lung to the brain and undergoes radiation therapy to the brain. Which of the following would be the principal diagnosis in this case?

    a. Ataxia

    b. Fractured arm

    c. Metastatic carcinoma of the brain

    d. Carcinoma of the lung

19. A patient was admitted for abdominal pain with diarrhea and was diagnosed with infectious gastroenteritis. The patient also has angina and chronic obstructive pulmonary disease. Which of the following would be the correct coding and sequencing for this case?

    a. Abdominal pain; infectious gastroenteritis; chronic obstructive pulmonary disease; angina

    b. Infectious gastroenteritis; chronic obstructive pulmonary disease; angina

    c. Gastroenteritis; abdominal pain; angina

    d. Gastroenteritis; abdominal pain; diarrhea; chronic obstructive pulmonary disease; angina

20. Patient has been diagnosed with acute major depression, sleep-related teeth grinding and psychogenic dysmenorrhea. The appropriate code assignment is:

    a. F32.81, F45.8

    b. F32.9, F45.89

    c. F32.9, F45.8, G47.63

    d. F32.9, G47.53

21. A patient is admitted with abdominal pain. The physician documents the discharge diagnosis as pancreatitis versus noncalculus cholecystitis. Both diagnoses are equally treated. The correct coding and sequencing for this case would be:

    a. Sequence either the pancreatitis or noncalculus cholecystitis as principal diagnosis

    b. Pancreatitis; noncalculus cholecystitis; abdominal pain

    c. Noncalculus cholecystitis; pancreatitis; abdominal pain

    d. Abdominal pain; pancreatitis; noncalculus cholecystitis

22. Which of the following developed the Diagnostic and Statistical Manual of Mental Disorders?

    a. Mental Health Association

    b. American Psychiatric Association

    c. Mental Health Foundation

    d. World Psychiatric Association

23. A seven-year-old patient was admitted to the emergency department for treatment of shortness of breath. The patient is given epinephrine and nebulizer treatments. The shortness of breath and wheezing are unabated following treatment. What diagnosis should be suspected?

    a. Acute bronchitis

    b. Acute bronchitis with chronic obstructive pulmonary disease

    c. Asthma with status asthmaticus

    d. Chronic obstructive asthma

24. A patient is seen in the emergency department for chest pain. After evaluation, it is suspected that the patient may have gastroesophageal reflux disease (GERD). The final diagnosis was "chest pain versus GERD." The correct ICD-10-CM code is:

    a. Z03.89, Encounter for observation for other suspected diseases and conditions ruled out

    b. R10.11, Right upper quadrant abdominal pain

    c. K21.9, Gastro-esophageal reflux disease

    d. R07.9, Chest pain, unspecified

25. A skin lesion is removed from a patient's cheek in the dermatologist's office. The dermatologist documents "skin lesion" in the health record. Before billing, the pathology report returns with a diagnosis of basal cell carcinoma. Which of the following actions should the coding professional do for claim submission?

    a. Code skin lesion

    b. Code benign skin lesion

    c. Code basal cell carcinoma

    d. Query the dermatologist

26. A 32-year-old woman in her 30th week of gestation is evaluated in her obstetrician's office for her second pregnancy with pre-existing essential hypertension. Assign the correct ICD-10-CM diagnostic code(s).

    a. O10.913, Z3A.31

    b. O10.919

    c. O10.412, Z3.40

    d. O10.013, Z3A.30

27. Which of the following purpose and use goals does *not* apply to ICD-10-PCS?

    a. Improved accuracy and efficiency of coding

    b. Reduced training effort

    c. Improved communication with physicians

    d. Improved collection of data about nursing care

28. When present, signs and symptoms that are *not* an integral part of the disease process:

    a. Should never be coded

    b. Should prompt a physician query

    c. Should be coded

    d. Should be coded with a Z-code

29. To help clarify terms that currently have overlapping meaning, ICD-10-PCS has defined root operations. What is an example of the root operation of Excision?

    a. Partial right nephrectomy

    b. Total nephrectomy

    c. Removal of left lung

    d. Complete mastectomy

30. The assignment of a diagnosis code is based on _____.

    a. The coding professional's assessment of the health record

    b. The provider's statement that the patient has a particular condition

    c. Clinical criteria used by the provider to establish the diagnosis

    d. Its inclusion in the discharge summary

31. A patient was discharged with the following diagnoses: "Cerebral artery occlusion, hemiparesis, and hypertension. The aphasia resolved before the patient was discharged." Which of the following code assignments would be appropriate for this case?

G81.90	Hemiplegia, unspecified affecting unspecified side
G81.91	Hemiplegia, unspecified affecting right dominant side
G81.92	Hemiplegia, unspecified affecting left dominant side
G81.93	Hemiplegia, unspecified affecting right nondominant side
G81.94	Hemiplegia, unspecified affecting left nondominant side
I66.9	Occlusion and stenosis of unspecified cerebral artery
I63.50	Cerebral infarction due to unspecified occlusion or stenosis of cerebral artery
I10	Hypertension
I50.9	Heart failure, unspecified
R47.01	Aphasia

   a. I63.50, G81.94, R47.01, I10
   b. I66.9, G81.90, R47.01, I10
   c. I66.9, G81.91, I10
   d. I66.9, G81.92, R47.01, I10

32. A patient is admitted to the hospital with shortness of breath and congestive heart failure. The patient subsequently develops respiratory failure. The patient undergoes intubation with ventilator management. Which of the following would be the correct sequencing and coding of this case?

   a. Congestive heart failure, respiratory failure, ventilator management
   b. Respiratory failure, intubation, ventilator management
   c. Respiratory failure, congestive heart failure, intubation, ventilator management
   d. Shortness of breath, congestive heart failure, respiratory failure, ventilator management

33. A physician correctly prescribes Coumadin. The patient takes the Coumadin as prescribed but develops hematuria as a result of taking the medication. Which of the following is the correct way to code this case?

   a. Poisoning due to Coumadin
   b. Unspecified adverse reaction to Coumadin
   c. Hematuria; poisoning due to Coumadin
   d. Hematuria; adverse reaction to Coumadin

34. A patient is admitted for chest pain with cardiac dysrhythmia to Hospital A. The patient is found to have an acute ST elevation (STEMI) inferior myocardial infarction with atrial fibrillation. After the atrial fibrillation was controlled and the patient was stabilized, the patient was transferred to Hospital B for a CABG × 3. Coumadin therapy and monitoring for the atrial fibrillation continued at Hospital B. Using the codes listed here, what are the appropriate ICD-10-CM codes and sequencing for both hospitalizations?

I21.09	ST elevation (STEMI) myocardial infarction involving other coronary artery of anterior wall
I21.19	ST elevation (STEMI) myocardial infarction involving other coronary artery of inferior wall
I22.0	Subsequent ST elevation (STEMI) myocardial infarction of anterior wall
I22.1	Subsequent ST elevation (STEMI) myocardial infarction of inferior wall
I48.0	Paroxysmal atrial fibrillation
I48.20	Chronic atrial fibrillation
I48.91	Unspecified atrial fibrillation
R07.9	Chest pain, unspecified
021209W	Bypass Coronary Artery, Three Arteries from Aorta with Autologous Venous Tissue, Open Approach

   a. Hospital A: I48.91, R07.9, I21.19; Hospital B: I22.1, I48.91, 021209W
   b. Hospital A: I21.09, I48.0; Hospital B: I22.0, I48.20, 021209W
   c. Hospital A: I21.19, I48.91; Hospital B: I21.19, I48.91, 021209W
   d. Hospital A: I21.19, I48.91; Hospital B: I22.1, I48.91, 021209W

35. A patient was admitted to the hospital with symptoms of a stroke and secondary diagnoses of COPD and hypertension. The patient was subsequently discharged from the hospital with a principal diagnosis of cerebral vascular accident and secondary diagnoses of catheter-associated urinary tract infection, COPD, and hypertension. Which of the following diagnoses should *not* be tagged as POA?

   a. Catheter-associated urinary tract infection
   b. Cerebral vascular accident
   c. COPD
   d. Hypertension

36. A 65-year-old female was admitted to the hospital. She was diagnosed with sepsis secondary to *Staphylococcus aureus* and abdominal pain secondary to diverticulitis of the colon. What is the correct code assignment?

   a. A41.89, K57.92, R10.9
   b. A41.01, K57.92
   c. A41.89, K57.92, A49.01
   d. A41.9, K57.92

37. Patient had carcinoma of the anterior bladder wall fulgurated three years ago. The patient returns yearly for a cystoscopy to recheck for bladder tumor. Patient is currently admitted for a routine check. A small recurring malignancy is found and fulgurated during the cystoscopy procedure. Which is the correct code assignment?

    a. C67.3, Z85.51, 0T5B8ZZ, 0TJB8ZZ

    b. C79.11, 0T5B8ZZ

    c. C67.3, 0T5B8ZZ

    d. C79.11, C67.3, 0T5B8ZZ

38. For the body mass index (BMI), depth of non-pressure chronic ulcers, pressure ulcer stage, coma scale, and NIH stroke scale (NIHSS) codes, code assignment may be based on the documentation provided by:

    a. Clinicians who are not the patient's provider (namely, physician or other qualified healthcare practitioner legally accountable for establishing the patient's diagnosis)

    b. The attending physician's documentation only

    c. The consulting physician's report

    d. The history and physical report from the attending surgeon

39. These codes are used to assign a diagnosis to a patient who is seeking health services but is not necessarily sick.

    a. C codes

    b. E codes

    c. M codes

    d. Z codes

40. The 38-year-old patient has an open reduction of a dislocation of the temporomandibular joint on the right side. The ICD-10-PCS code for this procedure is:

    a. 0RQC4ZZ

    b. 0RSD0ZZ

    c. 0RWC04Z

    d. 0RSC0ZZ

41. Assign the correct CPT code for the following procedure: Reposition of the pacemaker electrode.

    a. 33226

    b. 33243

    c. 33217

    d. 33215

42. Medicare requires a(n) _____ to identify a wound closed with tissue adhesives.

    a. Level II HCPCS code

    b. CPT code from the Repair section

    c. Modifier with the assigned HCPCS code

    d. E/M code

43. Patient returns during a 90-day postoperative period from a ventral hernia repair, now complaining of eye pain. What modifier would a physician setting use with the Evaluation and Management (E/M) code?

    a. -79, Unrelated procedure or service by the same physician during the postoperative period

    b. -25, Significant, separately identifiable evaluation and management service by the same physician on the same day of the procedure or other service

    c. -22, Increased procedural services

    d. -24, Unrelated evaluation and management service by the same physician during a postoperative period

44. A patient is admitted to an acute-care hospital for alcohol abuse and uncomplicated alcohol withdrawal syndrome due to chronic alcoholism. His blood alcohol level on admission was 10 mg/100 mL.

    a. F10.230, F10.10, Y90.0

    b. F10.230

    c. F10.10, Y90.0

    d. F10.230, Y90.0

45. A 45-year-old female is admitted for blood loss anemia due to dysfunctional uterine bleeding.

    a. D50.0, N93.8

    b. D62, N93.8

    c. N93.8, D50.0

    d. D50.0, D25.9

46. Patient admitted with left senile cortical cataract, diabetes mellitus, and extracapsular cataract extraction with simultaneous insertion of synthetic intraocular lens, via percutaneous approach.

    a. H25.012, E11.36, 08DK3ZZ, 08RK3JZ

    b. E11.9, H25.012

    c. E11.9, H25.092

    d. H25.012, E11.36, 08RK3JZ

47. A patient is admitted with acute exacerbation of COPD, chronic renal failure, and hypertension.

    a. J44.1, J44.9, I12.9, N18.9

    b. J44.1, N18.9, I10

    c. J44.9, N18.9, I10

    d. J44.1, I12.9, N18.9

48. Code only a confirmed diagnosis of Zika virus (A92.5, Zika virus disease) as documented by the provider. In this context, confirmation _____.

    a. Does not require documentation of the type of test performed; the physician's diagnostic statement that the condition is confirmed is sufficient

    b. Requires the documentation of the type of test in addition to the physician's diagnostic statement

    c. Must be provided by the laboratory findings report

    d. Requires that the public health agency be contacted

49. The four-year-old patient had an inguinal reducible herniorrhaphy. Assign the appropriate CPT code.

    a. 49495

    b. 49500

    c. 49505

    d. 49491

50. Identify the two-digit modifier that may be reported to indicate a physician performed the postoperative management of a patient, but another physician performed the surgical procedure.

    a. -22

    b. -54

    c. -32

    d. -55

51. What is the correct CPT code assignment for destruction of internal hemorrhoids with use of infrared coagulation?

    a. 46255

    b. 46930

    c. 46260

    d. 46945

52. Assign the level of medical decision-making: The 24-year-old patient was seen in the emergency department after an automobile accident. She complained of pain in her back and right leg. X-rays, UA, CBC were all normal. Discharge diagnosis: Thoracic/rib cage strain and contusion. Right leg contusion. She was discharged on Voltaren 50 mg three times a day for pain and Robaxin 750 mg three times a day for muscle spasms. She is told to return to work in a few days and to follow up with her family physician as necessary.

    a. Straightforward

    b. Low complexity

    c. Moderate complexity

    d. High complexity

53. The patient was admitted with major depression current episode severe, recurrent. What is the correct ICD-10-CM diagnosis code assignment for this condition?

    a. F33.2

    b. F33.40

    c. F32.9

    d. F31.81

54. A 35-year-old male was admitted with heartburn that has not improved with over-the-counter medications. An esophagoscopy and closed esophageal biopsy at the upper esophagus was performed. The physician documented esophageal reflux with esophagitis as the final diagnosis based on pathological examination. Identify the correct diagnosis and procedure codes.

    a. K23, 0DJ07ZZ

    b. K20.90, 0DB58ZX

    c. K21.00, 0DB18ZX

    d. K21.91, 0DB18ZX

55. Patient with flank pain was admitted and found to have calculi of both kidneys. A ureteroscopy with placement of bilateral ureteral stents was performed to expand the lumens so the stones could pass naturally. Assign the correct ICD-10-CM and ICD-10-PCS diagnosis and procedure codes.

    a. N20.0, N23, 0T788DZ

    b. N23, N20.0, 0TC68ZZ, 0TC78ZZ

    c. N20.0, 0T768DZ, 0T778DZ

    d. N20.0, 0T788DZ

56. A female patient is admitted for stress incontinence. A urethral suspension to reposition the urethra via open approach is performed. Assign the correct ICD-10-CM diagnosis and procedure codes.

    a. N39.3, 0TJB8ZZ

    b. N23, 0TSD0ZZ

    c. N39.3, 0TSD0ZZ

    d. R32, 0TSD4ZZ

57. Reference codes 49491 through 49525 for inguinal hernia repair. Patient is 47 years old. What is the correct code for an initial inguinal herniorrhaphy for incarcerated hernia?

    a. 49496

    b. 49501

    c. 49507

    d. 49521

58. If the documentation in a medical record does not indicate the type of diabetes but does indicate that the patient uses insulin, _____.

    a. Assign code E10, Type 1 diabetes mellitus

    b. Assign code E11, Type 2 diabetes mellitus

    c. Query the endocrinologist or attending physician

    d. Check the physician orders or medical order record for additional information

59. What is the correct CPT code assignment for hysteroscopy with lysis of intrauterine adhesions?

    a. 58555, 58559

    b. 58559

    c. 58559, 58740

    d. 58555, 58559, 58740

60. The physician performs an exploratory laparotomy with bilateral salpingo-oophorectomy. What is the correct CPT code assignment for this procedure?

    a. 49000, 58940, 58700

    b. 58940, 58720-50

    c. 49000, 58720

    d. 58720

61. Identify the CPT code for a 42-year-old diagnosed with ESRD who requires home dialysis for the month of April.

    a. 90965

    b. 90964

    c. 90966

    d. 90970

62. The patient presented to the physical therapy department and received 30 minutes of water aerobics therapeutic exercise with the therapist for treatment of arthritis. What is the appropriate treatment code(s) or modifier for a Medicare patient on a physical therapy plan of care in an outpatient setting?

    a. 97113

    b. 97113-50

    c. 97113, 97113

    d. 97110

63. Select the appropriate CPT code(s) to report a therapeutic subcutaneous injection of rabies immune globulin performed under direct physician supervision.

    a. 96372

    b. 90471

    c. 90375, 96372

    d. 90375, 90473

64. Identify the CPT procedure code for partial right-sided thyroid lobectomy with isthmusectomy and subtotal resection of left thyroid.

    a. 60210

    b. 60225

    c. 60220

    d. 60212

65. The patient presented in the ED with severe abdominal pain, amenorrhea. Serum human chorionic gonadotropin (hCG) was lower than normal. There were also endometrial and uterine changes. Patient diagnosed with right tubal pregnancy. A laparoscopic removal of tubal pregnancy, right side, was performed. Which of the following is the correct code assignment?

    a. O00.80, 10T24ZZ, 0UT54ZZ

    b. O00.101, 10T24ZZ

    c. O00.109, 10T24ZZ

    d. O00.109, 0UT54ZZ

66. The patient, a 47-year-old male with a protracted history of urinary retention due to benign prostatic hyperplasia, is being treated in the outpatient surgery suite. The urologist inserts an endoscope in the penile urethra and dilates the structure to allow instrument passage. After endoscope placement, a radiofrequency stylet is inserted, and the diseased prostate is excised with radiant energy. Bleeding is controlled with electrocoagulation. Following instrument removal, a catheter is inserted and left in place. Which of the following code sets will be reported for this service?

    a. N40.1, R33.8, 53852

    b. N40.0, 52601

    c. D29.1, 53852

    d. N40.3, R33.9, 53850

67. Identify the CPT procedure code(s) and correct modifier(s) for a screening mammogram and a diagnostic mammogram performed on a patient on the same day.

    a. 77067-GH

    b. 77067, 77066-GG

    c. 77066-GG

    d. 77065, 77053-GH

Domain 2 *Reimbursement Methodologies*

68. Given the following information, which of the following statements is correct?

	MCD	Type	MS-DRG Title	Weight	Discharges	Geometric Mean	Arithmetic Mean
191	04	MED	Chronic obstructive pulmonary disease w CC	0.9757	10	4.1	5.0
192	04	MED	Chronic obstructive pulmonary disease w/o CC/MCC	0.7254	20	3.3	4.0
193	04	MED	Simple pneumonia & pleurisy w MCC	1.4327	10	5.4	6.7
194	04	MED	Simple pneumonia & pleurisy w CC	1.0056	20	4.4	5.3
195	04	MED	Simple pneumonia & pleurisy w/o CC/MCC	0.7316	10	3.5	4.1

    a. In each MS-DRG the geometric mean is lower than the arithmetic mean.

    b. In each MS-DRG the arithmetic mean is lower than the geometric mean.

    c. The higher the number of patients in each MS-DRG, the greater the geometric mean for that MS-DRG.

    d. The geometric means are lower in MS-DRGs that are associated with a CC or MCC.

69. If another status T procedure were performed, how much would the facility receive for the second status T procedure?

Billing Number	Status Indicator	CPT/HCPCS	APC
998323	V	99285-25	0612
998324	T	25500	0044
998325	X	72050	0261
998326	S	72128	0283
998327	S	70450	0283

   a. 0%

   b. 50%

   c. 75%

   d. 100%

70. Determining medical necessity for inpatient services does not always include:

   a. Local coverage determinations

   b. Related monetary benefits to payers

   c. Uniform written procedures for appeals

   d. Concurrent review

71. Which of the following types of hospitals are excluded from the Medicare inpatient prospective payment system?

   a. Children's hospitals

   b. Rural hospitals

   c. State-supported hospitals

   d. Tertiary hospitals

72. The MS-DRGs are organized into:

   a. Case-mix classifications

   b. Geographic practice cost indices

   c. Major diagnostic categories

   d. Resource-based relative values

73. The Medicare program pays for healthcare services, Social Security benefits for those age 65 and older, permanently disabled people, and those with:

   a. End-stage renal disease

   b. Military experience

   c. Medicaid

   d. Skilled nursing services

74. Which of the following is *not* reimbursed according to the Medicare outpatient prospective payment system?

    a. Community Mental Health Center (CMHC) partial hospitalization services

    b. Critical access hospitals

    c. Hospital outpatient departments

    d. Vaccines provided by Comprehensive Outpatient Rehabilitation Facilities (CORF)

75. Fee schedules are updated by third-party payers:

    a. Annually

    b. Monthly

    c. Semiannually

    d. Weekly

76. Which of the following would a health record technician use to perform the billing function for a physician's office?

    a. CMS-1500

    b. UB-04

    c. UB-92

    d. CMS 1450

77. When a provider accepts assignment, this means the:

    a. Patient authorizes payment to be made directly to the provider

    b. Provider agrees to accept as payment in full the allowed charge from the fee schedule

    c. Balance billing is allowed on patient accounts, but at a limited rate

    d. Participating provider receives a fee-for-service reimbursement

78. A coding audit shows that an inpatient coding professional is using multiple codes that describe the individual components of a procedure rather than using a single code that describes all the steps of the procedure performed. Which of the following should be done in this case?

    a. Require all coding professionals to implement this practice

    b. Report the practice to the Office of Inspector General (OIG)

    c. Counsel the coding professional and stop the practice immediately

    d. Put the coding professional on unpaid leave of absence

79. Prospective payment systems were developed by the federal government to:

    a. Increase healthcare access

    b. Manage Medicare and Medicaid costs

    c. Implement managed care programs

    d. Eliminate fee-for-service programs

80. Given NCCI edits, if the placement of an infusion catheter is billed along with the performance of an infusion procedure for the same date of service for an outpatient beneficiary, Medicare will pay for:

    a. The placement of the catheter

    b. The placement of the catheter and the infusion procedure

    c. The infusion procedure

    d. Neither the placement of the catheter nor the infusion procedure

81. The goal of coding compliance programs is to reduce:

    a. Liability in regards to fraud and abuse

    b. Delays in claims processing

    c. Billing errors

    d. Inaccurate code assignments

82. Which of the following actions would be best to determine whether present on admission (POA) indicators for the conditions selected by CMS are having a negative impact on the hospital's Medicare reimbursement?

    a. Identify all records for a period having these indicators for these conditions and determine if these conditions are the only secondary diagnoses present on the claim that will lead to higher payment.

    b. Identify all records for a period that have these indicators for these conditions.

    c. Identify all records for a period that have these indicators for these conditions and determine whether or not additional documentation can be submitted to Medicare to increase reimbursement.

    d. Take a random sample of records for a period of time for records having these indicators for these conditions and extrapolate the negative impact on Medicare reimbursement.

83. From the information provided, how many APCs would this patient have?

Billing Number	Status Indicator	CPT/HCPCS	APC
998323	V	99285-25	0612
998324	T	25500	0044
998325	X	72050	0261
998326	S	72128	0283
998327	S	70450	0283

    a. 1

    b. 4

    c. 5

    d. 3

84. If a patient's total outpatient bill and allowable is $500, and the patient's healthcare insurance plan pays 80 percent of the allowable charges, what is the amount owed by the patient?

    a. $10

    b. $40

    c. $100

    d. $400

85. In a managed fee-for-service arrangement, which of the following would be used as a cost-control process for inpatient surgical services?

    a. Prospectively pre-certify the necessity of inpatient services

    b. Determine what services can be bundled

    c. Audit all inpatient claims on an annual basis

    d. Require the patient to pay 20 percent of the inpatient bill

86. The sum of a hospital's total relative MS-DRG weights for a year was 15,192 and the hospital had 10,471 total discharges for the year. Given this information, what would be the hospital's case-mix index for that year?

    a. 0.6896

    b. 1.5901

    c. 1.45×100

    d. 1.4500

87. In processing a bill under the Medicare outpatient prospective payment system (OPPS) in which a patient had three surgical procedures performed during the same operative session, which of the following would apply?

    a. Bundling of services

    b. Outlier adjustment

    c. Pass-through payment

    d. Discounting of procedures

88. The government sponsored supplemental medical insurance that covers physician and surgeon services, emergency department, outpatient clinic, labs and physical therapy is:

    a. Medicaid

    b. Medicare Part B

    c. Medicare Part A

    d. Medicare Part D

89. A denial of a claim is possible for all of the following reasons *except*:

    a. Not meeting medical necessity

    b. Billing too many units of a specific service

    c. Unbundling

    d. Approved precertification

90. Promoting correct coding and control of inappropriate payments is the basis of NCCI claims processing edits that help identify claims not meeting medical necessity. The NCCI automated prepayment edits used by payers is based on all of the following *except*:

    a. Coding conventions defined in the CPT book

    b. National and local policies and coding edits

    c. Analysis of standard medical and surgical practice

    d. Clinical documentation in the discharge summary

91. The NCCI editing system used in processing OPPS claims is referred to as:

    a. Outpatient code editor (OCE)

    b. Outpatient national editor (ONE)

    c. Outpatient perspective payment editor (OPPE)

    d. Outpatient claims editor (OCE)

92. Denials of outpatient claims are often generated from all of the following edits *except*:

    a. National Correct Coding Initiative (NCCI)

    b. Outpatient code editor (OCE)

    c. Outpatient claims editor (OCE)

    d. National and local policies

93. Timely and correct reimbursement is dependent on:

    a. Adjudication

    b. Clean claims

    c. Remittance advice

    d. Actual charge

94. Solutions to address the problem of dirty claims include all of the following *except*:

    a. Submitting paper claims

    b. Submitting claims electronically

    c. Using electronic health record system that eliminates manual or duplicate entry of data

    d. Auditing claims' accuracy and compliance with edits prior to submitting

95. Which of the following is *not* an essential data element for a healthcare insurance claim?

    a. Revenue code

    b. Procedure code

    c. Provider name

    d. Procedure name

96. CMS has made significant advances to link quality to reimbursement using _____ programs, which provide accountability by healthcare providers.

    a. Value-based purchasing (VBP)

    b. Cost-based reimbursement (CBR)

    c. Pay for performance design (PPD)

    d. Prospective payment system (PPS)

97. The pre-MDC assignment for MS-DRGs is based on:

    a. The principal diagnosis

    b. Admission diagnosis

    c. A defined set of ICD-10-PCS procedures

    d. The primary procedure

98. The government-sponsored program that provides expanded coverage of many healthcare services including HMO plans, PPO plans, special needs plans, and Medical Savings accounts is:

    a. Medicare Advantage

    b. Medicare Part A

    c. Medicare Part B

    d. Medigap

99. When clean claims are submitted, they can be adjudicated in many ways through computer software automatically. Which statement is *not* one of the outcomes that can occur as part of auto-adjudication?

    a. Auto-pay

    b. Auto-suspend

    c. Auto-calculate

    d. Auto-deny

100. What system assigns each service a value representing the true resources involved in producing it, including the time and intensity of work, the expenses of practice, and the risk of malpractice?

    a. MS-DRGs

    b. RVUs

    c. CPT

    d. HCPCS

101. What statement is *not* reflective of meeting medical necessity requirements?

    a. A service or supply provided for the diagnosis, treatment, cure, or relief of a health condition, illness, injury, or disease.

    b. A service or supply provided that is not experimental, investigational, or cosmetic in purpose.

    c. A service provided that is necessary for and appropriate to the diagnosis, treatment, cure, or relief of a health condition, illness, injury, disease, or its symptoms.

    d. A service provided solely for the convenience of the insured, the insured's family, or the provider.

102. A patient has two health insurance policies: Medicare and a Medicare supplement. Which of the following statements is true?

    a. The patient receives any monies paid by the insurance companies over and above the charges.

    b. Coordination of benefits is necessary to determine which policy is primary and which is secondary so that there is no duplication of payments.

    c. The decision on which company is primary is based on remittance advice.

    d. The patient should not have a Medicare supplement.

103. What system reimburses hospitals a predetermined amount for each Medicare inpatient admission?

    a. APR-DRG

    b. MS-DRG

    c. APC

    d. RUG

104. What is one way that physicians can prevent or minimize potentially abusive or fraudulent activities?

    a. Developing a compliance plan

    b. Upcoding

    c. Unbundling

    d. Billing for noncovered services

105. The MS-DRG system creates a hospital's case-mix index (types or categories of patients treated by the hospital) based on the relative weights of the MS-DRG. The case mix can be figured by multiplying the relative weight of each MS-DRG by the number of _____ within that MS-DRG.

    a. Admissions

    b. Discharges

    c. CCs

    d. MCCs

106. Medicare beneficiaries who have low incomes and limited financial resources may also receive assistance from which federal matching program?

    a. Social Security

    b. Medicare Advantage

    c. Tricare

    d. Medicaid

107. Under the OPPS, on which code set is the APC system primarily based for outpatient procedures and services including devices, drugs, and other covered items?

    a. CPT/HCPCS

    b. ICD-10-CM

    c. CDT

    d. MS-DRG

108. Sometimes hospital departments must work together to solve claims issue errors to prevent them from happening repeatedly. What departments would need to work together if an audit found that the claim did not contain the procedure code or charge for a pacemaker insertion?

    a. Health Information and Business Office

    b. Health Information, Materials Management, and Cardiac Department

    c. Health Information, Business Office, and Cardiac Department

    d. Health Information and Radiology

109. Which of the following best describes the type of coding utilized when a CPT/HCPCS code is assigned directly through the charge description master for claim submission and bypasses the record review and code assignment by the facility coding staff?

    a. Hard coding

    b. Soft coding

    c. Encoder coding

    d. Natural-language processing coding

110. In 2004, as part of HHS, CMS implemented _____ to provide fair and accurate payments while rewarding efficiency and high-quality care for Medicare's chronically ill population.

    a. Accountable care organizations (ACOs)

    b. Hierarchical condition categories (CMS-HCCs)

    c. Value-based care

    d. Expanded prospective payment system (PPS)

111. A patient is admitted to the hospital with abdominal pain. The principal diagnosis is cholecystitis. The patient also has a history of hypertension and diabetes. In the MS-DRG prospective payment system, which of the following would determine the major diagnostic category (MDC) assignment for this patient?

    a. Abdominal pain

    b. Cholecystitis

    c. Hypertension

    d. Diabetes

112. Which of the following is a condition that arises during hospitalization?

    a. Case mix

    b. Complication

    c. Comorbidity

    d. Principal diagnosis

113. Identify where the following information would be found in the acute-care record: "CBC: WBC 12.0, RBC 4.65, HGB 14.8, HCT 43.3, MCV 93."

    a. Medical laboratory report

    b. Pathology report

    c. Physical examination

    d. Physician orders

114. Identify where the following information would be found in the acute-care record: "PA and Lateral Chest: The lungs are clear. The heart and mediastinum are normal in size and configuration. There are minor degenerative changes of the lower thoracic spine."

    a. Medical laboratory report

    b. Physical examination

    c. Physician progress note

    d. Radiography report

115. The following is documented in an acute-care record: "Microscopic: Sections are of squamous mucosa with no atypia." Where would this documentation be found?

    a. History

    b. Pathology report

    c. Physical examination

    d. Operation report

116. The following is documented in an acute-care record: "Admit to 3C. Diet: NPO. Meds: Compazine 10 mg IV Q 6 PRN." Where would this documentation be found?

    a. Physician order

    b. History

    c. Physical examination

    d. Progress notes

117. What is the primary use of the case-mix index?

    a. Benchmark of emergency department levels

    b. Defines how a hospital compares to peers and whether the facility is at risk

    c. Audit of APCs and the comparison to same-size hospitals

    d. Tool for the coding manager to compare coding professional productivity

Domain 3 *Health Records and Data Content*

118. Which of the following elements is *not* a component of most patient records?

    a. Patient identification

    b. Clinical history

    c. Financial information

    d. Test results

119. Identify where the following information would be found in the acute-care record: "Following induction of an adequate general anesthesia, and with the patient supine on the padded table, the left upper extremity was prepped and draped in the standard fashion."

    a. Anesthesia report

    b. Physician progress notes

    c. Operative report

    d. Recovery room record

120. The following is documented in an acute-care record: "38 weeks gestation, Apgars 8/9, 6# 9.8 oz, good cry." Where would this documentation be found?

    a. Admission note

    b. Clinical laboratory

    c. Newborn record

    d. Physician order

121. The following is documented in an acute-care record: "Atrial fibrillation with rapid ventricular response, left axis deviation, left bundle branch block." Where would this documentation be found?

    a. Admission order

    b. Clinical laboratory report

    c. ECG report

    d. Radiology report

122. The following is documented in an acute-care record: "Spoke to the attending re: my assessment. Provided adoption and counseling information. Spoke to CPS re: referral. Case manager to meet with patient and family." Where would this documentation be found?

    a. Admission note

    b. Nursing note

    c. Physician progress note

    d. Social work note

123. Deidentified data are used for:

    a. Patient care

    b. Education of healthcare staff

    c. Public health and research

    d. Development of policies and procedures

124. Even though state laws may be more stringent, CMS requires acute healthcare records to be maintained by the acute healthcare organization for:

    a. Ten years

    b. At least five years

    c. Minimum of 25 years

    d. Permanent access

125. A notation for a diabetic patient in a physician progress note reads: "Occasionally gets hungry. No insulin reactions. Says she is following her diabetic diet." In which part of a POMR progress note would this notation be written?

    a. Subjective

    b. Objective

    c. Assessment

    d. Plan

126. A notation for a diabetic patient in a physician progress note reads: "FBS 110 mg%, urine sugar, no acetone." In which part of a POMR progress note would this notation be written?

    a. Subjective

    b. Objective

    c. Assessment

    d. Plan

127. A notation for a hypertensive patient in a physician ambulatory care progress note reads: "Continue with Diuril, 500 mgs once daily. Return visit in 2 weeks." In which part of a POMR progress note would this notation be written?

    a. Subjective

    b. Objective

    c. Assessment

    d. Plan

128. A notation for a hypertensive patient in a physician ambulatory care progress note reads: "Blood pressure adequately controlled." In which part of a POMR progress note would this notation be written?

   a. Subjective

   b. Objective

   c. Assessment

   d. Plan

129. Reviewing the health record for missing signatures, missing medical reports, and ensuring that all documents belong in the health record is an example of _____ review.

   a. Quantitative

   b. Qualitative

   c. Statistical

   d. Outcomes

130. Which of the following terms means that data should be complete, accurate, and consistent?

   a. Data privacy

   b. Data confidentiality

   c. Data integrity

   d. Data safety

131. The admitting data of Mrs. Smith's health record indicated that her birth date was March 21, 1948. On the discharge summary, Mrs. Smith's birth date was recorded as July 21, 1948. Which quality element is missing from Mrs. Smith's health record?

   a. Data completeness

   b. Data consistency

   c. Data accessibility

   d. Data comprehensiveness

132. Which of the following is an example of clinical data?

   a. Admitting diagnosis

   b. Date and time of admission

   c. Insurance information

   d. Health record number

133. Documentation of aides who assist a patient with activities of daily living, bathing, laundry, and cleaning would be found in which type of specialty record?

   a. Home health

   b. Behavioral health

   c. End-stage renal disease

   d. Rehabilitative care

134. Which of the following materials is *not* documented in an emergency care record?

    a. Patient's instructions at discharge

    b. Time and means of the patient's arrival

    c. Patient's complete medical history

    d. Emergency care administered before arrival at the facility

135. Which of the following provides macroscopic and microscopic information about tissue removed during an operative procedure?

    a. Anesthesia report

    b. Laboratory report

    c. Operative report

    d. Pathology report

136. What is the defining characteristic of an integrated health record format?

    a. Each section of the record is maintained by the patient care department that provided the care.

    b. Integrated health records are intended to be used in ambulatory settings.

    c. Integrated health records include both paper forms and computer printouts.

    d. Integrated health record components are arranged in strict chronological order.

137. Which of the following represents documentation of the patient's current and past health status?

    a. Physical examination

    b. Medical history

    c. Physician orders

    d. Patient consent

138. Which of the following is a goal of a CDI program?

    a. Analyze the records after the patient is discharged to document the missing pieces of information

    b. Identify and clarify missing, conflicting, or nonspecific physician documentation related to diagnoses and procedures

    c. Identify the providers who are not performing procedures

    d. Ensure that the documentation is meeting the minimum requirements set by the medical staff bylaws

139. What is the function of a consultation report?

    a. Provides a chronological summary of the patient's medical history and illness

    b. Documents opinions about the patient's condition from the perspective of a physician not previously involved in the patient's care

    c. Concisely summarizes the patient's treatment and stay in the hospital

    d. Documents the physician's instructions to other parties involved in providing care to a patient

140. What is the function of physician's orders?

    a. Provide a chronological summary of the patient's illness and treatment

    b. Document the patient's current and past health status

    c. Document the physician's instructions to other parties involved in providing care to a patient

    d. Document the provider's follow-up care instructions given to the patient or patient's caregiver

141. In the acute-care facility, the patient identity management tool that ensures that the right patient connects to the right information relies on:

    a. Master patient index (MPI)

    b. Case-mix index (CMI)

    c. The organization's clinical staff guidelines

    d. Cancer registry

142. Medicare defines fraud as _____.

    a. Billing practices that are inconsistent with generally acceptable fiscal policies

    b. Making unintentional billing errors

    c. Accurately representing the types of services provided, dates of services, or identity of the patient

    d. Intentional deception or misrepresentation that results in an unauthorized benefit to an individual

143. Which governmental agency develops an annual work plan that delineates the specific target areas for Medicare that will be monitored in a given year?

    a. Centers for Medicare and Medicaid (CMS)

    b. Federal Bureau of Investigation (FBI)

    c. Office of Inspector General (OIG)

    d. Defense Criminal Investigative Service (DCIS)

144. The physician comes into the HIM department and requests the HIM director to pull all of his records from the previous year in which the principal diagnosis of myocardial infarction was indicated. Where would the HIM director begin to pull these records?

    a. Disease index

    b. Master patient index

    c. Operative index

    d. Physician index

145. Identify the acute-care record report where the following information would be found: "Set up appointment at the Hypertension Center. Hold potassium supplements. Phenergan p.o. 12.5 mg 1–2 tablets p.o. prn every 6 hrs."

    a. Medical laboratory report

    b. Pathology report

    c. Physical exam

    d. Physician order

146. The attending physician is responsible for which of the following types of acute-care documentation?

    a. Consultation report

    b. Discharge summary

    c. Laboratory report

    d. Pathology report

Domain 4   *Compliance*

147. In a joint effort of the Department of Health and Human Services (HHS), Office of Inspector General (OIG), Centers for Medicare and Medicaid Services (CMS), and Administration on Aging (AOA), which program was released in 1995 to target fraud and abuse among healthcare providers?

    a. Operation Restore Trust

    b. Medicare Integrity Program

    c. Tax Equity and Fiscal Responsibility Act (TEFRA)

    d. Medicare and Medicaid Patient and Program Protection Act

148. All of the following should be part of the core areas of a coding compliance plan *except*:

    a. Physician query process

    b. Correct use of encoder software

    c. Coding diagnoses supported by medical record documentation

    d. Tracking length of stay

149. Common forms of fraud and abuse include all of the following *except*:

    a. Upcoding

    b. Unbundling or "exploding" charges

    c. Refiling claims after denials

    d. Billing for services not furnished to patients

150. Which of the following is considered the most innocent of improper payments because there is no intent to falsely receive a payment from the payer?

    a. Fraud

    b. Abuse

    c. Mistake

    d. Unbundling

151. To combat fraud and abuse in coding, one strategy is to:

    a. Use computer-assisted coding (CAC)

    b. Unbundle codes

    c. Use best practices to write a query to clarify documentation

    d. Implement the meaningful use incentive program

152. Using uniform terminology is a way to improve:

    a. Validity

    b. Data timeliness

    c. Audit trails

    d. Data reliability

153. The _____ mandated the development of standards for electronic medical records.

    a. Medicare and Medicaid legislation of 1965

    b. Prospective Payment Act of 1983

    c. Health Insurance Portability and Accountability Act (HIPAA) of 1996

    d. Balanced Budget Act of 1997

154. Messaging standards for electronic data interchange in healthcare have been developed by:

    a. HL7

    b. IEE

    c. Joint Commission

    d. CMS

155. The privacy officer reports breaches to the Office of Civil Rights in the Department of Health and Human Services. Which of the following breach notification statements is correct?

    a. The privacy officer must notify the Secretary of Health and Human Services.

    b. The privacy officer must report breaches of both secured and unsecured PHI.

    c. The privacy officer must report a breach to the Board of Directors of the organization.

    d. Breach notification applies only when 20 or more individuals are affected.

156. A valid authorization must contain all of the following *except*:

    a. A description of the information to be used or disclosed

    b. A signature and stamp by a notary

    c. A statement that the information being used or disclosed may be subject to redisclosure by the recipient

    d. An expiration date or event

157. A record of all transactions in the computer system that is maintained and reviewed for unauthorized access is called a(n) _____.

    a. Security breach

    b. Audit trail

    c. Unauthorized access

    d. Privacy trail

158. The _____ permits penalties to be awarded to those who intentionally submit fraudulent claims to the US government.

    a. Anti-kickback statute

    b. Balanced Budget act of 1997

    c. False Claims Act

    d. Health Insurance Portability and Accountability Act of 1996

159. Performance counseling usually begins with which of the following?

    a. Submitting an action plan of steps the employee will do to resolve the issue and improve performance

    b. Job termination

    c. Informal counseling or verbal warning

    d. Putting the coding professional on unpaid leave of absence

160. A health information technician (HIT) is hired as the chief compliance officer for a large group practice. In evaluating the current program, the HIT learns that there are written standards of conduct and policies and procedures that address specific areas of potential fraud as well as audits in place to monitor compliance. Which of the following should the compliance officer also ensure are in place?

    a. Compliance program education and training programs for all employees in the organization

    b. Establishment of a hotline to receive complaints and adoption of procedures to protect whistleblowers from retaliation

    c. Adoption of procedures to adequately identify individuals who make complaints so that appropriate follow-up can be conducted

    d. Establishment of a corporate compliance committee that reports directly to the CFO

161. In developing a coding compliance program, which of the following would not be ordinarily included as participants in coding compliance education?

    a. Current coding personnel

    b. Medical staff

    c. Newly hired coding personnel

    d. Nursing staff

162. Which of the following issues compliance program guidance?

    a. AHIMA

    b. CMS

    c. Federal Register

    d. OIG

163. The practice of assigning a diagnosis or procedure code specifically for the purpose of obtaining a higher level of payment is called _____.

    a. Billing

    b. Unbundling

    c. Upcoding

    d. Unnecessary service

164. The Charge Description Master coordinator tasks include planning for a review of payment system rules and:

    a. Verification of CDI compliance within the CDM

    b. Incorporation of CMS rule changes into the CDM

    c. Ensuring clinical staff approval for the CDM update

    d. Updating the organization's policies and procedures relevant to the CDM

165. In 2009, HHS and the DOJ created the _____ to prevent waste, fraud and abuse, reduce healthcare costs, and improve the quality of care provided to Medicare patient.

    a. Office of Inspector General (OIG)

    b. Recovery Audit Contractor (RAC)

    c. Quality Improvement Organization and Enforcement (QIO)

    d. Health Care Fraud Prevention Team (HEAT)

166. Identify the two types of queries used in clinical documentation integrity:

    a. Electronic and computer-assisted

    b. Manual and computer-assisted

    c. Manual and electronic

    d. Paper and electronic

167. An intentional misrepresentation that an individual knows to be false and knowing that the act could result in some unauthorized benefit to some other person is an example of:

    a. Abuse

    b. Ethical behavior

    c. Fraud

    d. Scam

168. In developing a coding compliance program, which of the following would not be ordinarily included as participants in coding compliance education?

    a. Current coding personnel

    b. Medical staff

    c. Newly hired coding personnel

    d. Nursing staff

169. Which of the following personnel should be authorized, per hospital policy, to take a physician's verbal order for the administration of medication?

    a. Unit secretary working on the unit where the patient is located

    b. Nurse working on the unit where the patient is located

    c. Health information director

    d. Admissions registrars

170. The Medicare Modernization Act (MMA) of 2003 called for CMS to launch a Medicare payment recovery demonstration project. The purpose of the act eventually resulted in the implementation of a group contracted by the government to monitor suspicious and improper activity of Medicare payments including overpayments and underpayments. What is this group?

    a. Operation Restore Trust

    b. Payment Error Prevention Program

    c. Recovery audit contractors

    d. Medicare administrative contractors

Domain 5 *Information Technologies*

171. The quality control function for the EHR that shows the format in which the data will be displayed is the:

    a. Unit numbering system

    b. Input mask

    c. Drop down option

    d. Checkbox

172. Computer software programs that assist in the assignment of codes used with diagnostic and procedural classifications are called _____.

    a. Natural-language processing systems

    b. Monitoring or audit programs

    c. Encoders

    d. Concept, description, and relationship clinical decision support

173. Which of the following is used by some healthcare organizations to extract information for research and reimbursement purposes from an electronic health record?

    a. Integrated workflow processes

    b. Computer-assisted coding

    c. Electronic document management system

    d. Speech recognition system

174. Computer-assisted coding may use _____, which means that digital text from online documents stored in the information system is read directly by the software, which then suggests codes to match the documentation.

    a. Encoded vocabulary

    b. Natural-language processing

    c. Data exchange standards

    d. Structured reports

175. An encoder that is built using expert system techniques such as rule-based systems is a(n):

    a. Encoder interface

    b. Logic-based encoder

    c. Automated code book encoder

    d. Grouper

176. The communication and network technologies connections, known as _____, are used by providers to submit orders for medications and lab tests.

    a. Computerized order entry systems (CPOEs)

    b. Bar code medication administration records (BC-MARs)

    c. Electronic health records (EHRs)

    d. Personal health record (PHRs)

177. Which of the following make data entry easier but may harm data quality?

    a. Use of templates

    b. Copy and paste

    c. Drop-down boxes

    d. Structured data

178. Which decision support system could deliver a reminder to a physician that it is time for the patient's flu shot?

    a. Document-driven

    b. Executive

    c. Clinical

    d. Management

179. The HIM department is planning to scan medical record documentation. The project includes the scanning of documentation such as history and physicals, physician orders, operative reports, and nursing notes. Which of the following methods of scanning would be best to help HIM professionals monitor the completeness of health records during a patient's hospitalization?

    a. Ad hoc

    b. Concurrent

    c. Retrospective

    d. Post discharge

180. The patient's address is the same in the master patient index, electronic health record, laboratory information system, and other information systems. This means that the data values are consistent and therefore indicative of which of the following?

    a. Data availability

    b. Data integrity

    c. Data privacy

    d. Data accessibility

Domain 6 | *Confidentiality and Privacy*

181. What is the legal term used to define the protection of health information in a patient–provider relationship?

    a. Access

    b. Confidentiality

    c. Privacy

    d. Security

182. Which of the following is an advance directive created by an individual, while still competent, that designates another person (proxy) to make his or her healthcare decisions consistent with the individual's wishes on his or her behalf?

    a. Do-not-resuscitate order

    b. Durable power of attorney for healthcare decisions (DPOA-HCD)

    c. Informed consent

    d. Living will

183. Which of the following is a direct command that requires an individual or a representative of an organization to appear in court or to present an object to the court?

    a. Judicial decision

    b. Subpoena

    c. Credential

    d. Regulation

184. The term *minimum necessary* means that healthcare providers and other covered entities must limit use, access, and disclosure to the minimum necessary to _____.

    a. Satisfy one's curiosity

    b. Accomplish the intended purpose

    c. Treat an individual

    d. Perform research

185. The number that has been proposed for use as a unique patient identification number but is controversial because of confidentiality and privacy concerns is the _____.

    a. Social security number

    b. Unique physician identification number

    c. Health record number

    d. National provider identifier

186. Which of the following is *not* true of the Notices of Privacy Practices?

    a. It must be made available at the site where the individual is treated.

    b. It must be posted in a prominent place.

    c. It must contain content that may not be changed.

    d. It must be prominently posted on the covered entity's website when the entity has one.

187. Section 4004 of the _____ defines practices that constitute information blocking and authorized the HHS Secretary to identify reasonable and necessary activities that do not constitute information blocking, or exceptions.

    a. 21st Century Cures Act

    b. Patient Protection and Affordable Care Act (ACA)

    c. Omnibus Budget Reconciliation Act

    d. Healthcare Quality Improvement Act

188. The Information Governance Principles for Healthcare (IGPHC) includes the statement that, "An organization shall maintain its information for an appropriate time, taking into account its legal, regulatory, fiscal, operational, risk, and historical requirements." Identify the principle.

    a. Principle of Protection

    b. Principle of Integrity

    c. Principle of Accountability

    d. Principle of Retention

189. What is the process used to transform text into an unintelligible string of characters that can be transmitted via communications media with a high degree of security and then decrypted when it reaches a secure destination?

    a. Distortion

    b. Extrication

    c. Encryption

    d. Encoded

190. Which of the following is true regarding the HIPAA Privacy Rule and fundraising?

    a. Fundraising materials do not have to include opt-out instructions.

    b. Prior authorization is required if individuals are not targeted based on diagnosis.

    c. Authorization is always required for fundraising solicitations.

    d. Individuals must be informed in the Notice of Privacy Practices that their information may be used for fundraising purposes.

191. Which of the following is true regarding HIPAA security provisions?

    a. Covered entities must appoint two chief security officers who can share security responsibilities for 24-hour coverage.

    b. Covered entities must conduct employee security training sessions every six months for all employees.

    c. Covered entities must retain policies for six years after they are no longer in effect.

    d. Covered entities must conduct technical and nontechnical evaluations every six years.

192. Which of the following statements is true of the Notice of Privacy Practices?

    a. It gives the covered entity permission to use information for treatment purposes.

    b. It gives the covered entity permission to use information for TPO purposes.

    c. It must be provided to every individual at the first time of contact or service with the covered entity.

    d. It must be provided to the individual by the covered entity within 30 days after receipt of treatment or service.

193. Online transaction processing is conducted in which of the following?

    a. Clinical data repository

    b. Clinical data warehouse

    c. Data analytics system

    d. Online analytical processor

194. A special webpage that offers secure access to data is called a(n) _____.

    a. Access control

    b. Home page

    c. Intranet

    d. Portal

195. The _____ was issued by the Office of the National Coordinator (ONC) for health information technology to be a resource to the nation as a vision and reference.

    a. Health Information Technology for Economic and Clinical Health (HITECH)

    b. American Recovery and Reinvestment Act (ARRA)

    c. Meaningful Use (MU) program

    d. Federal Health Information Technology Strategic Plan 2015–2020

196. Data definition refers to:

    a. Meaning of data

    b. Completeness of data

    c. Consistency of data

    d. Detail of data

197. The filing system that distributes health records evenly throughout the filing system is:

    a. Terminal digit

    b. Alphanumeric

    c. Straight numeric

    d. Alphabetic

198. This system requires the author to sign into the system using a user ID and password to complete the entries made:

    a. Digital dictation

    b. Electronic signature authentication

    c. Encoder

    d. Clinical data repository

199. Coding professionals will assign codes that have been selected into a computer program called a(n) _____ to assign the patient's case to the correct group based on ICD-10-CM/PCS or CPT/HCPCS codes.

    a. Encoder

    b. MPI

    c. Natural-language processor

    d. Grouper

200. A threat to data security is:

    a. Encryption

    b. Malware

    c. Audit trail

    d. Data quality

EXAM 1

Domain 1 *Clinical Classification Systems*

1. Identify the ICD-10-CM code for a patient with a subsequent encounter for routine healing of a closed traumatic capital epiphyseal fracture of the left femur.

   a. S79.012A

   b. S79.019D

   c. M84.452D

   d. S79.012D

2. Identify the ICD-10-CM code(s) for neonatal tooth eruption.

   a. K01.1

   b. K00.6, K08.0

   c. K01.0

   d. K00.6

3. Identify CPT code(s) for the following patient. A 35-year-old female undergoes an excision of a 3.0-cm tumor in her forehead. An incision is made through the skin and subcutaneous tissue. The tumor is dissected free of surrounding structures. The wound is closed with interrupted sutures.

   a. 21012

   b. 21012, 12052

   c. 21014

   d. 21014, 12052

4. Identify CPT code(s) for the following Medicare patient. A 67-year-old female undergoes an excision of a breast lesion identified by preoperative placement of radiological marker.

   a. 19101

   b. 19101, 19125

   c. 19125

   d. 19125, 19126

5. Identify the ICD-10-CM codes for an open skull fracture with subarachnoid and subdural hemorrhage, expired due to brain injury without regaining consciousness, initial encounter.

   a. S02.80XB, S06.4X7A S06.5X7A

   b. S02.81XB, S06.5X7A

   c. S06.6X7A, S06.5X7A, S06.4X7A

   d. S02.91XB, S06.6X7A, S06.5X7A

6. Identify the ICD-10-PCS codes for insertion of dual chamber cardiac pacemaker battery via an incision in the subcutaneous tissue of the chest wall, and percutaneous transvenous insertion of right atrial and right ventricular leads.

   a. 0JH606Z, 02H73JZ, 02HL3JZ

   b. 0WH80YZ, 02H63JZ, 02HK3JZ

   c. 0WH80YZ, 02H73JZ, 02HL3JZ

   d. 0JH606Z, 02H63JZ, 02HK3JZ

7. Identify the correct ICD-10-PCS code for thrombectomy of arteriovenous dialysis graft. The operative report indicates that the AV graft is located in the right upper arm with the right cephalic vein being obstructed with the thrombus. An incision was performed as the approach.

   a. 05DD0ZZ

   b. 05FD3ZZ

   c. 05CD0ZZ

   d. 05BD0ZX

8. Identify the appropriate ICD-10-CM code(s) for Mobitz type I and II heart block.

   a. I44.7, I45.19

   b. I44.1

   c. I45.0, I45.2

   d. I45.10

9. Identify the appropriate ICD-10-CM and ICD-10-PCS codes for cardiac pacemaker pulse generator check.

   a. Z45.010, 4B02XSZ

   b. Z45.018, 4B02XTZ

   c. T82.121A, 4B02XSZ

   d. Z45.010, 4B02XTZ

10. When both hypertension and a condition classifiable to category N18, Chronic kidney disease (CKD), are present, assign codes from category:

    a. I13, Hypertensive heart and chronic kidney disease

    b. I15, Secondary hypertension

    c. I12, Hypertensive chronic kidney disease

    d. I27.0, Primary pulmonary hypertension

11. Identify the appropriate ICD-10-PCS code(s) for a coronary artery bypass of two sites, one using the left internal mammary artery to the left proximal anterior descending artery, and one using the right internal mammary artery to the distal left anterior descending artery, both done via thoracotomy.

    a. 02104K8, 02104K9

    b. 02110A8, 02110A9

    c. 02100Z8, 02100Z9

    d. 021109W

12. Coronary arteriography serves as a diagnostic tool in detecting obstruction within the coronary arteries. Identify the technique using two catheters inserted percutaneously through the femoral artery.

    a. Brachial

    b. Stones

    c. Judkins

    d. Femoral

13. Identify the correct ICD-10-CM code(s) for a patient who arrives at the hospital for outpatient laboratory services ordered by the physician to monitor the patient's Coumadin levels.
A prothrombin time (PT) is performed to check the patient's long-term use of his anticoagulant treatment.

    a. Z51.81, Z79.01

    b. Z51.81, Z79.02

    c. Z79.01, R79.1

    d. Z79.01

14. The patient was admitted to the outpatient department for a diagnostic procedure. An endoscope was inserted through the anus and advanced to the transverse colon. The procedure was stopped due to poor prep. Assign the physician's service for this procedure.

    a. 45384

    b. 45378-53

    c. 45378

    d. 45346-52

15. Identify the CPT code(s) for the following patient: A two-year-old boy presented to the hospital to have his gastrostomy tube repositioned under fluoroscopic guidance.

    a. 43752

    b. 43761

    c. 43761, 76000

    d. 49450

16. Identify the ICD-10-CM code(s) for the following: threatened abortion with hemorrhage at 15 weeks; home undelivered.

    a. O20.0, O20.9

    b. O20.0, Z3A.15

    c. O20.8

    d. O20.8, Z3A.15

17. Identify the ICD-10-CM code for diaper rash in elderly patient.

    a. L21.9

    b. L22

    c. R21

    d. L74.3

18. For ulcers that were present on admission but healed at the time of discharge, assign the code for the site and stage of the pressure ulcer _____.

    a. According to the discharge condition

    b. According to the nursing progress notes

    c. According to the condition at time of admission

    d. As documented in the discharge summary

19. Identify the ICD-10-CM code for anaphylactic shock due to ingestion of pecans, initial encounter.

    a. T78.01XA

    b. T78.05XA

    c. T78.1XXA

    d. T78.09XA

20. Identify the ICD-10-CM code(s) for acute osteomyelitis of the right index finger due to *Staphylococcus aureus*.

    a. M86.142

    b. M86.149, B95.61

    c. M86.141, A49.01

    d. M86.141, B95.61

21. For a new patient, the physician documents a moderate level of complexity, a limited data review, and moderate risk. Which E/M code should be assigned?

    a. 99214

    b. 99204

    c. 99203

    d. 99202

22. Identify the ICD-10-CM code(s) for other specified aplastic anemia secondary to adverse effect of chemotherapy, subsequent encounter.

    a. D61.2

    b. D61.1, T45.1X5D

    c. D64.9

    d. D63.0, T45.1X5D

23. Identify the ICD-10-CM code(s) for the following: A six-month-old child is scheduled for a clinic visit for a routine well-child examination. The physician documents, "well child, born premature."

    a. Z00.00, P07.30

    b. Z00.129

    c. Z00.129, P07.30

    d. Z00.129, O60.10X0

24. Identify the chapter of ICD-10-CM in which certain signs and symptoms of breast disease, such as mastodynia, induration of breast, and nipple discharge, are included.

    a. Chapter 2: Neoplasms

    b. Chapter 12: Diseases of the Skin and Subcutaneous Tissue

    c. Chapter 14: Diseases of the Genitourinary System

    d. Chapter 18: Symptoms, Signs and Abnormal Clinical and Laboratory Findings, Not Elsewhere Classified

25. Devices used as part of the procedure and removed as the procedure concludes _____ assigned the ICD-10-PCS sixth character.

    a. Are

    b. Are not

    c. Can be

    d. Are often

26. If a patient is admitted with a pressure ulcer at one stage and it progresses to a higher stage, the coding professional should:

    a. Assign two separate code—one code for the site and stage of the ulcer on admission and a second code for the same ulcer site and the highest stage reported during the stay.

    b. Assign only the highest stage documented during the stay.

    c. Assign only the stage of the ulcer on admission.

    d. Query the attending physician for the appropriate site and stage of the pressure ulcer.

27. Identify the correct ICD-10-PCS code(s) for laparoscopic cholecystectomy. The entire gallbladder was removed.

    a. 0FT40ZZ

    b. 0FT40ZZ, 0FJ44ZZ

    c. 0FT44ZZ, 0FJ44ZZ

    d. 0FT44ZZ

28. The 67-year-old male patient was admitted with a significant pleural effusion and congestive heart failure. The physician performed a thoracentesis. Later that same day, the patient's lungs again filled with fluid; the same physician performed a second thoracentesis. Which of the following is the correct code assignment for the physician or hospital?

    a. 32551

    b. 32554, 32554-76

    c. 32554-27

    d. 32601, 32650-78

29. What is the best reference tool to determine how CPT codes should be assigned?

    a. Local coverage determination from Medicare

    b. American Medical Association's *CPT Assistant* newsletter

    c. American Hospital Association's *Coding Clinic*

    d. Centers for Medicare and Medicaid Services website

30. A 71-year-old male was discharged with primary osteoarthritis of the left hip. He underwent a total replacement of his left hip, with ceramic-bearing surface, cemented. How are the diagnosis and procedure coded?

    a. M16.12, 0SRB039

    b. M16.0, 0SRB01A

    c. M16.9, 0SW90JZ

    d. M16.11, 0SP90JZ

31. Which of the following software applications would be used to aid in the coding function in a physician's office?

    a. Grouper

    b. Encoder

    c. Pricer

    d. Diagnosis calculator

32. In fiscal year 2008, Medicare revamped the inpatient payment system to incorporate three severity levels. The grouping is known as:

    a. AP-DRGs

    b. RBRVS

    c. MS-DRGs

    d. APR-DRGs

33. The healthcare program for active duty members of the military and other qualified family members is:

    a. Children's Health Insurance Program (CHIP)

    b. Veterans Insurance

    c. Tricare

    d. Workers' compensation

34. An electrolyte panel (80051) in the Laboratory section of CPT consists of tests for carbon dioxide (82374), chloride (82435), potassium (84132), and sodium (84295). If each of the component codes are reported and billed individually on a claim form, this would be a form of:

    a. Optimizing

    b. Unbundling

    c. Sequencing

    d. Classifying

35. In the Laboratory section of CPT, if a group of tests overlaps two or more panels, report the panel that incorporates the greatest number of tests to fulfill the code definition. What would a coding professional do with the remaining test codes that are not part of a panel?

    a. Report the remaining tests using individual test codes, according to CPT.

    b. Do not report the remaining individual test codes.

    c. Report only those test codes that are part of a panel.

    d. Do not report a test code more than once regardless of whether the test was performed twice.

36. The Office of Inspector General's (OIG) Compliance Program for Hospitals recommends that hospitals appoint a chief compliance officer and:

    a. Establish a compliance committee

    b. Report their case mix annually

    c. Monitor the fraud hotline

    d. Assign CDI professionals to audit claims

37. The front end of the revenue cycle management process does not include:

    a. Enterprise-wide scheduling system

    b. Claims appeals

    c. Order tracking system

    d. Financial function system

38. What is the best reference tool for ICD-10-CM and ICD-10-PCS coding advice?

    a. CMS Inpatient Prospective Payment System (IPPS)

    b. ICD-10-CM and ICD-10-PCS Coding Guidelines

    c. AHA's *Coding Clinic for ICD-10-CM/PCS*

    d. National Correct Coding Initiative (NCCI)

39. CMS developed medically unlikely edits (MUEs) to prevent providers from billing units of services greater than the norm would indicate. These MUEs were implemented on January 1, 2007, and are applied to which code set?

    a. ICD-10-PCS codes

    b. HCPCS/CPT codes

    c. ICD-10-CM codes

    d. LOINC

40. Several key principles require appropriate physician documentation to secure payment from the insurer. Which of the following fails to impact payment based on physician responsibility?

    a. The health record should be complete and legible.

    b. The rationale for ordering diagnostic and other ancillary services should be documented or easily inferred.

    c. The charges and services should be documented on the itemized bill.

    d. The patient's progress and response to treatment and any revision in the treatment plan and diagnoses should be documented.

41. Which of the following does *not* need to be included in the documentation of each patient encounter to secure payment from the insurer?

    a. The reason for the encounter and the patient's relevant history, physical examination, and prior diagnostic test results

    b. A patient assessment, clinical impression, or diagnosis

    c. A plan of care

    d. The identity of the patient's nearest relative and emergency contact number

42. Two Medicare patients were hospitalized with bacterial pneumonia. One patient was hospitalized for three days, and the other patient was hospitalized for 30 days. Both cases result in the same MS-DRG with different lengths of stay. Which of the following most closely describes how the hospital will be reimbursed?

    a. The hospital will receive the same MS-DRG for both patients but additional reimbursement will be allowed for the patient who stayed 30 days because the length of stay was greater than the geometric length of stay for this MS-DRG.

    b. The hospital will receive the same reimbursement for the same MS-DRG regardless of the length of stay.

    c. The hospital can appeal the payment for the patient who was in the hospital for 30 days because the cost of care was significantly higher than the average length of stay for the MS-DRG payment.

    d. The hospital will receive a day outlier for the patient who was hospitalized for 30 days.

43. Which classification system is in place to reimburse home health agencies?

    a. MS-DRGs

    b. PDPM

    c. HHRGs

    d. APCs

44. On October 1, 2012, the Affordable Care Act established which of the following, requiring CMS to reduce payments to IPPS hospitals with excess admissions?

    a. Hospital-acquired conditions (HACs)

    b. MS-DRGs

    c. Hospital Readmissions Reduction Program

    d. RUG-III

45. The CMS-HHC model indicates the cost of the individual relative to the average beneficiary through a measure identified as the:

    a. Case mix

    b. Risk score

    c. Major diagnostic category

    d. Resource-based relative value

46. Which of the following types of hospitals are excluded from the Medicare acute-care prospective payment system?

    a. Children's hospitals

    b. Small, community hospitals

    c. Tertiary hospitals

    d. Trauma hospitals

47. CMS identified conditions that are not present on admission and could be "reasonably preventable." Hospitals are not allowed to receive additional payment for these conditions when the condition is present on admission. What are these conditions called?

    a. Conditions of Participation

    b. Not present on admission

    c. Hospital-acquired conditions

    d. Hospital-acquired infections

48. Which of the following fails to meet the CMS classification of a hospital-acquired condition?

    a. Foreign object retained after surgery

    b. Air embolism

    c. Gram-negative pneumonia

    d. Blood incompatibility

49. The focus on the delivery, measurement, and provision of quality patient care led to several initiatives that link reimbursement to quality care. These initiatives are referred to as:

    a. Audits and claim denials

    b. Never events

    c. Value-base purchasing

    d. Ethical executive programs

50. The maximum number of Ambulatory Payment Classifications (APCs) that may be reported per outpatient encounter is:

    a. One

    b. Six

    c. Ten

    d. No maximum number

51. Each code in the HCPCS has been assigned a(n) _____ that establishes how a service, procedure, or item is paid in OPPS.

    a. Payment Status Indicator (SI)

    b. Outpatient Code Editor (OCE)

    c. Medicare Summary Notice (MSN)

    d. Remittance advice (RA)

52. An addendum to the health record should be dated:

    a. The day that the error was identified

    b. The day the care provided occurred

    c. The day the addendum was created

    d. The day the patient was discharged

53. The seven characteristics of high-quality documentation include clarity, completeness, consistency, legibility, preciseness, reliability, and:

    a. Regular auditing

    b. Processing

    c. Benchmarking

    d. Timeliness

54. The physician has signed a statement that all of her dictated reports should be automatically considered approved and signed unless she makes corrections within 72 hours of dictating. This is called:

    a. Auto-authentication

    b. Electronic signature

    c. Automatic record completion

    d. Chart tracking

Domain 3 *Health Records and Data Content*

55. When creating requirements of documentation for hospital bylaws, which of the following should be evaluated?

    a. The personal preferences of the healthcare practitioners

    b. The documentation needs based on accrediting bodies

    c. Information taught in the local nursing programs

    d. The wishes of the department staff

56. Which of the following is *not* a function of the discharge summary?

    a. Providing information about the patient's insurance coverage

    b. Ensuring the continuity of future care

    c. Providing information to support the activities of the medical staff review committee

    d. Providing concise information that can be used to answer information requests

57. Under HIPAA, at the time of admission to the facility or prior to treatment by the provider, patients must be informed about the use of individually identifiable health information by signing the:

    a. Patient consent form

    b. Notice of Privacy Practices

    c. Advance directives

    d. Advance Beneficiary Notice

58. A 65-year-old white male was admitted to the hospital on 1/15 complaining of abdominal pain. The attending physician requested an upper GI series and laboratory evaluation of CBC and UA. The x-ray revealed possible cholelithiasis, and the UA showed an increased white blood cell count. The patient was taken to surgery for an exploratory laparoscopy, and a ruptured appendix was discovered. The chief complaint was _____.

    a. Ruptured appendix

    b. Exploratory laparoscopy

    c. Abdominal pain

    d. Cholelithiasis

59. All documentation entered in the medical record relating to the patient's diagnosis and treatment is considered to be this type of data:

    a. Clinical

    b. Identification

    c. Secondary

    d. Financial

60. What type of data is exemplified by the insured party's member identification number?

    a. Demographic data

    b. Clinical data

    c. Certification data

    d. Financial data

61. Which of the following is the type of MPI matching algorithm that assigns weights to specific data elements and uses the weights to compare one record to another?

    a. Deterministic

    b. Rules-based

    c. Probabilistic

    d. Centralized

62. Two patients were assigned the same health record number. This is an example of a(n):

    a. Overlap

    b. Overlay

    c. Purge

    d. Duplicate

63. Mildred Smith was admitted from an acute-care hospital to a nursing facility with the following information: "Patient is being admitted for organic brain syndrome." Underneath the diagnosis, her medical information along with her rehabilitation potential was also listed. On which form is this information documented?

    a. Transfer or referral form

    b. Release of information form

    c. Patient rights acknowledgment

    d. Admitting physical evaluation

64. According to the Joint Commission Accreditation Standards, which document must be placed in the patient's record before a surgical procedure may be performed?

    a. Admission record

    b. Physician's order

    c. Report of history and physical examination

    d. Discharge summary

65. Bob Smith was admitted to Mercy Hospital on June 21. The physical examination was completed on June 23. According to Medicare Conditions of Participation, which statement applies to this situation?

    a. The record is not in compliance because the physical examination must be completed within 24 hours of admission.

    b. The record is not in compliance because the physical examination must be completed within 48 hours of admission.

    c. The record is in compliance because the physical examination must be completed within 48 hours of admission.

    d. The record is in compliance because the physical examination was completed within 72 hours of admission.

66. A health record with deficiencies that is not completed within the timeframe specified in the medical staff rules and regulations is called a(n):

    a. Suspended record

    b. Delinquent record

    c. Pending record

    d. Illegal record

67. The coding of clinical diagnoses and healthcare procedures and services after the patient is discharged is what type of review?

    a. Proactive

    b. Prospective

    c. Concurrent

    d. Retrospective

68. To comply with Joint Commission standards, the HIM director wants to ensure that history and physical examinations are documented in the patient's health record no later than 24 hours after admission. Which of the following would be the *best* way to ensure the completeness of health records?

    a. Retrospectively review each patient's health record to make sure history and physicals are present.

    b. Review each patient's health record concurrently to make sure history and physicals are present to meet accreditation standards.

    c. Establish a process to review health records immediately on discharge.

    d. Do a review of health records for all patients discharged in the previous 60 days.

69. Medical record completion compliance is a problem at Community Hospital. The number of incomplete charts often exceeds the standard set by the Joint Commission, risking a type I violation. Previous HIM committee chairpersons tried multiple methods to improve compliance, including suspension of privileges and deactivating the parking garage keycard of any physician in poor standing. To improve compliance, which of the following would be the next step to overcome noncompliance?

    a. Discuss the problem with the hospital CEO, CIO, and CFO.

    b. Call the Joint Commission.

    c. Contact other hospitals to see what methods they use to ensure compliance.

    d. Drop the issue because noncompliance is always a problem.

70. Reviewing the health record for missing signatures, missing medical reports, and ensuring that all documents belong in the health record is an example of what type of analysis?

    a. Quantitative

    b. Qualitative

    c. Statistical

    d. Outcomes

Domain 4 *Compliance*

71. How do accreditation organizations such as the Joint Commission use the health record?

    a. To serve as a source for case study information

    b. To determine whether the documentation supports the provider's claim for reimbursement

    c. To provide healthcare services

    d. To determine whether standards of care are being met

72. Valley High, a skilled nursing facility, wants to become certified to take part in federal government reimbursement programs such as Medicare. What standards must the facility meet in order to become certified for these programs?

    a. Joint Commission Accreditation Standards

    b. Accreditation Association for Ambulatory Healthcare Standards

    c. Conditions of Participation

    d. Outcomes and Assessment Information Set

73. An effective compliance program should include some basic elements to comply with state and federal laws. These include policies, procedures, and standards of conduct; the identification of a compliance officer and committee; education of staff; establishment of communication channels; performance of internal monitoring; corrective action when a problem is identified; and:

    a. Clinical documentation strategies

    b. Penalties for noncompliance of standards

    c. Improvement of the accuracy of health claims

    d. External audits

74. Identify which of the federal fraud and abuse laws prohibits a physician's referral of designated health services for Medicare and Medicaid patients if the physician has a financial relationship with the entity.

    a. False Claims Act

    b. Anti-Kickback Statute

    c. Stark Law

    d. HIPAA

75. Corporate compliance programs were released by the OIG for hospitals to develop and implement their own compliance programs. Which of the following is *not* a basic element of a corporate compliance program?

    a. Designation of a chief compliance officer

    b. Implementation of regular and effective education and training programs for all employees

    c. Designation of a medical staff appointee for documentation compliance

    d. The use of audits or other evaluation techniques to monitor compliance

76. Which of the following programs has been in place in hospitals for years and has been required by the Medicare and Medicaid programs and accreditation standards?

    a. Internal DRG audits

    b. Peer review

    c. Managed care

    d. Quality improvement

77. HIM coding professionals and the organizations that employ them have the responsibility to not tolerate behavior that adversely affects data quality. Which of the following is an example of behavior that should *not* be tolerated?

    a. Omit codes that reflect negatively on quality and patient safety measurement.

    b. Follow-up on and monitor identified problems.

    c. Evaluate and trend diagnoses and procedure code selections.

    d. Report data quality review results to organizational leadership, compliance staff, and the medical staff.

78. Two types of physician queries are:

    a. Open-ended and multiple-choice

    b. Paper and electronic

    c. Standardized and nonstandardized

    d. Inpatient and outpatient

79. Maintenance of the CDM requires expertise in coding, clinical procedures, health record or clinical documentation, and:

    a. Applicable software

    b. Billing regulations

    c. Claim denials

    d. Staffing changes

80. CDM software is primarily designed to continuously apply edits to point out compliance issues, check validity of CPT and revenue codes and:

    a. Identify item pricing

    b. Focus on payment rates

    c. Review potential CDI issues

    d. Regulate charges

81. Standardizing medical terminology to avoid differences in naming various medical conditions and procedures (such as the synonyms bunionectomy, McBride procedure, and repair of hallux valgus) is one purpose of _____.

    a. Transaction standards

    b. Content and structure standards

    c. Vocabulary standards

    d. Security standards

82. The inpatient CDI process can be divided into three main functions: query for documentation clarification, physician education, and:

    a. Record review

    b. Health record completion

    c. Quality improvement

    d. Coding productivity

83. For coding and billing professionals, being compliant means to perform one's job functions according to the laws, regulations, and guidelines with integrity as set forth by Medicare and other third-party payers. This is an example of:

    a. Ethics

    b. Skills

    c. Behaviors

    d. Education

Domain 5 *Information Technologies*

84. Which of the following describes the capability for two or more information systems to communicate and exchange information electronically?

    a. Sharing

    b. Interchange

    c. Mapping

    d. Interoperability

85. What software will prompt the user through a variety of questions and choices based on the clinical terminology entered to assist the coding professional in selecting the most appropriate code?

    a. Logic-based encoder

    b. Automated codebook

    c. Speech recognition software

    d. Natural-language processing

86. The technology commonly used for automated claims processing (sending bills directly to third-party payers) is _____.

    a. Optical character recognition

    b. Bar coding

    c. Neural networks

    d. Electronic data interchange

87. Which type of data entered into electronic systems is free text and has no specific requirements or rules for data entry?

    a. Unstructured data

    b. Structured data

    c. Formatted data

    d. Unformatted data

88. Although CAC is used mainly for coding of the health record for reimbursement, another purpose is:

    a. Auditing

    b. Queries

    c. CDI

    d. Utilization review

89. Dr. Smith dictated his report and then immediately edited it. What type of speech recognition is being used?

    a. Back-end

    b. Front-end

    c. Physician

    d. Outsourced

90. A standard vocabulary is used to achieve what type of interoperability?

    a. Process

    b. Semantic

    c. System

    d. Technical

Domain 6   *Confidentiality and Privacy*

91. A valid authorization requires which of the following?

    a. A statement that the Notice of Privacy Practices has been provided

    b. An expiration date or event

    c. A statement that patient understands his or her rights related to PHI

    d. A patient account number

92. Methods of authentication include smart cards, biometrics, and:

    a. Firewalls

    b. Digital certificates

    c. Passwords

    d. Encryption

93. The right of an individual to keep his or her personal information from being disclosed to anyone is a definition of:

    a. Confidentiality

    b. Privacy

    c. Integrity

    d. Security

94. The Final Rule that defines practices which constitute information blocking and authorizes the Secretary of Health and Human Services (HHS) to identify reasonable and necessary activities that do not constitute information blocking (referred to as "exceptions") is which of the following?

    a. Section 4004 of the 21st Century Cures Act

    b. Minimum Data Set for Long-Term Care

    c. Resident Assessment Protocol

    d. Outcomes and Assessment Information Set

95. Which of the following statements is true of the Notice of Privacy Practices?

    a. It gives the covered entity permission to use information for treatment purposes.

    b. It gives the covered entity permission to use information for treatment, payment and healthcare operations purposes.

    c. It must be provided to every individual at the first time of contact or service with the covered entity.

    d. It must be provided to the individual by the covered entity within 30 days after receipt of treatment or service.

96. The OIG believes that compliance programs have benefits in addition to submitting accurate claims. This includes all of the following *except* _____.

    a. Demonstration of the organization's commitment to be responsible for the conduct toward employees and the community

    b. Provision of a more accurate view of behavior relating to fraud and abuse

    c. Increased potential for criminal and unethical conduct

    d. Improvements in the quality of patient care

97. The factors to be considered with destruction of records include applicable federal and state statutes and regulations, accreditation standards, pending or ongoing litigation, cost, and:

    a. Patient advocacy

    b. Authorization requirements

    c. Storage capabilities

    d. Strategic planning

98. What does an audit trail check for?

    a. Unauthorized access to a system

    b. Loss of data

    c. Presence of a virus

    d. Successful completion of a backup

99. An individual designated as an inpatient coding professional may have access to an electronic health record to code the record. Under what access security mechanism is the coding professional allowed access to the system?

    a. Role-based

    b. User-based

    c. Context-based

    d. Situation-based

100. In what form of health information exchange are data centrally located but physically separated?

    a. Consolidated

    b. Consolidated federated

    c. Centralized

    d. Federated

EXAM 2

Domain 1 *Clinical Classification Systems*

1. Identify the correct ICD-10-CM diagnosis code(s) and sequencing for the following: patient seen in the medical clinic with a scar on the right hand secondary to a laceration sustained two years ago.

    a. L90.5

    b. S61.411S

    c. L90.5, S61.411S

    d. S61.411S, L90.5

2. Report the correct CPT code(s) for the following procedure: a malignant lesion is excised and the resultant skin defect is closed with a Z-plasty.

    a. Assign the code for the Z-plasty only (14000–14061).

    b. Assign the code for the malignant lesion excision (11600–11646) and a code for the Z-plasty (14000–14061).

    c. Assign the code for the complex repair only (13100–13160).

    d. Assign the code for the malignant lesion excision only (11600–11646).

3. Identify the correct ICD-10-CM diagnosis code(s) for the following: patient suffered a partial traumatic metacarpophalangeal amputation of his right index and middle fingers.

    a. S68.011A, S68.012A

    b. S68.120A, S68.122A

    c. S68.011D, S68.012D

    d. S68.011S

4. The qualifier used in the ICD-10-PCS code for root operation Bypass indicates:

    a. Origin of bypass

    b. Nothing, the qualifier 2 is assigned

    c. The body part bypassed to

    d. The type of stent used to form the bypass

5. Identify the correct ICD-10-CM diagnosis code(s) for a patient with near-syncope event and nausea.

    a. R55

    b. R55, R11.0

    c. R55, R11.2

    d. R42, R11.0

6. Identify the correct ICD-10-CM diagnosis code(s) for a patient with an elevated glucose tolerance test.

    a. R73.9

    b. R73.01

    c. R73.01, R73.9

    d. R73.02

7. The patient underwent a vaginal delivery with internal version at 40 weeks. Identify the correct ICD-10-PCS code.

   a. 10D07Z7

   b. 10D07Z3

   c. 10D00Z1

   d. 10D07Z6

8. Identify the correct ICD-10-CM diagnosis code(s) for a patient with seizures; epilepsy ruled out.

   a. R56.9

   b. G40.901

   c. R56.9, G40.909

   d. G40.909

9. Identify the correct ICD-10-CM diagnosis code for a male patient with stress urinary incontinence.

   a. N39.46

   b. R32

   c. N39.3

   d. N39.498

10. Identify the correct ICD-10-CM diagnosis code(s) for a patient hospitalized and treated for vancomycin-resistant sepsis requiring treatment.

    a. A49.01

    b. A41.2, Z16.30

    c. A41.9, Z16.21

    d. Z16.30, A41.02

11. Identify the punctuation mark that is used to supplement words or explanatory information that may or may not be present in the statement of a diagnosis in ICD-10-CM coding. The punctuation does not affect the code number assigned to the case and is considered a nonessential modifier.

    a. Parentheses ( )

    b. Square brackets [ ]

    c. Slanted brackets *[ ]*

    d. Braces { }

12. The hierarchy for CPT code 47100, Biopsy of the liver (wedge), is: Surgery, Digestive System, Liver, _____, Code

    a. Excision

    b. Incision

    c. Drainage

    d. Repair

13. When a patient is seen by a new or different provider over the course of treatment for a pathological fracture, assignment of the seventh character is based on whether _____.

    a. The patient is undergoing active treatment

    b. The provider is seeing the patient for the first time

    c. Routine healing occurs

    d. There is a complication in the healing process (namely, malunion, nonunion, sequelae)

14. Identify the correct ICD-10-CM diagnosis codes for metastatic carcinoma of the colon to the left lung.

    a. C18.9, C34.92

    b. C78.00, C18.9

    c. C18.9, C78.02

    d. C18.9, D49.1

15. When a procedure is commonly carried out with another procedure, it may be designated as a(n):

    a. Modifier

    b. Add-on code

    c. Category I code

    d. Category III code

16. Identify the ICD-10-CM diagnosis code(s) for poorly controlled type 2 diabetes mellitus; mild malnutrition.

    a. E11.65, E46

    b. E10.65, E44.1

    c. E11.65, E44.1

    d. E10.65, E46

17. Identify the ICD-10-PCS code for the following procedure: right kidney transplant, organ donor match.

    a. 0TR30KZ

    b. 0TS00ZZ

    c. 0TY00Z0

    d. 0TW507Z

18. Identify the correct E/M codes for the following day of care: the physician sees a patient in his office in the morning and then again in the afternoon at which time he sends the patient to the hospital for observation status. Later that same day, he visits the patient in the hospital and admits him as a full inpatient.

    a. Assign two E/M codes for the office visits, one for observation care and one for the inpatient admission.

    b. Assign one code for the observation care and one code for the inpatient admission.

    c. Assign one code for the inpatient admission only.

    d. Assign one code to combine the two office visits, one code for the observation care and one for the inpatient admission.

19. Category II codes cover all but one of the following topics. Which is *not* addressed by Category II codes?

    a. Patient management

    b. New technology

    c. Therapeutic, preventative, or other interventions

    d. Patient safety

20. Per CPT guidelines, services reported separately are:

    a. Coded when performed as part of another, larger procedure

    b. Specifically identifiable, performed on the same date of another E/M service

    c. Never coded under any circumstance

    d. Only appropriate when approved by the provider by means of a coding query

21. Dr. Whitteker performed a total abdominal hysterectomy with removal of fallopian tubes and ovaries. Dr. Salmon provided the surgical assistance. Which CPT code(s) should be assigned for this case?

    a. 58150

    b. 58575, 58575-81

    c. 58150, 58150-80

    d. 58550, 58552

22. The codes in the musculoskeletal section of CPT may be used by _____.

    a. Orthopedic surgeons only

    b. Orthopedic surgeons and emergency department physicians

    c. Any physician

    d. Orthopedic surgeons and neurosurgeons

23. Observation E/M codes (99218–99220) are used in physician billing when _____.

    a. A patient is admitted and discharged on the same date

    b. A patient is admitted for routine nursing care following surgery

    c. A patient does not meet admission criteria

    d. A patient is referred to a designated observation status

24. Documentation of the history of use of drugs, alcohol, and tobacco is part of the _____.

    a. Past medical history

    b. Social history

    c. Systems review

    d. History of present illness

25. Tissue transplanted from one individual to another of the same species, but different genotype is called a(n) _____.

    a. Autograft

    b. Xenograft

    c. Allograft graft

    d. Heterograft

26. If an orthopedic surgeon attempted to reduce a fracture but was unsuccessful in obtaining acceptable alignment, what type of code should be assigned for the procedure?

    a. A "with manipulation" code

    b. A "without manipulation" code

    c. An unlisted procedure code

    d. An E/M code only

27. Discharge services provided to a normal newborn, admitted and discharged on the same day, are assigned to code _____.

    a. 99238

    b. 99460

    c. 99239

    d. 99463

28. In coding arterial catheterizations, _____ is when the tip of the catheter is manipulated from the insertion into the aorta and then out into another artery.

    a. Selective catheterization

    b. Nonselective catheterization

    c. Manipulative catheterization

    d. Radical catheterization

29. Which element(s) are *not* required for assignment of the MS-DRG?

    a. Diagnoses and procedures (principal and secondary)

    b. Attending and consulting physicians

    c. Presence of major or other complications and comorbidities (MCC or CC)

    d. Discharge disposition or status

30. Which of the following statements about Category III CPT codes is *false*?

    a. They are updated only once every two years.

    b. They were developed to reflect emerging technologies and procedures.

    c. They are archived after five years if the code has not been accepted for inclusion in the main body of CPT.

    d. Reimbursement for these services is dependent on individual payer policy.

31. The patient is a 45-year-old female who fell while walking her dog. She was walking on the sidewalk in her neighborhood and accidently tripped and subsequently fell. She sustained a comminuted fracture of the shaft of her right tibia confirmed by x-ray done in the emergency room. She also hit her head on a fire hydrant and suffered a slight concussion but no loss of consciousness. The patient also had a splinter of wood in her elbow from the fall. The patient was admitted and taken to surgery, where an open reduction with internal fixation was accomplished with good alignment of fracture fragments. Post-op course was uneventful, and the patient was discharged with daily physical therapy at home. What is the appropriate code assignment?

    a. S82.251A, S06.0X0A, S50.359A, W01.198A, Y92.480, Y93.K1, Y99.8, 0QSG04Z

    b. S82.252A, S06.0X0A, W01.198A, Y92.481, Y93.K1, Y99.8, 0QSG06Z

    c. S82.253A, S06.0X0A, S50.359A, W01.198A, Y92.480, Y93.K1, Y99.8, 0QSG34Z

    d. S82.254A, S06.0X0A, W01.190A, Y92.482, Y93.K1, Y99.8, 0QSH04Z

Domain 2   *Reimbursement Methodologies*

32. How does Medicare or other third-party payers determine whether the patient has medical necessity for the tests, procedures, or treatment billed on a claim form?

    a. By requesting the medical record for each service provided

    b. By reviewing all the diagnosis codes assigned.

    c. By reviewing all physician orders

    d. By reviewing the discharge summary and history and physical report.

33. What is the name of the organization that develops the billing form that hospitals are required to use?

    a. American Academy of Billing Forms (AABF)

    b. National Uniform Billing Committee (NUBC)

    c. National Uniform Claims Committee (NUCC)

    d. American Billing and Claims Academy (ABCA)

34. Each HCPCS code has been assigned a(n) _____ that establishes how a service, procedure, or item is paid in OPPS.

    a. Payment status indicator (SI)

    b. Ambulatory Payment Classification (APC)

    c. Outpatient Code Editor (OCE)

    d. Cost-to-charge ration (CCR)

35. The goal of the MS-DRG system is to improve Medicare's capability to recognize _____.

    a. Severity of illness in its inpatient hospital payments

    b. Poor quality of care and reimburse hospitals based on performance

    c. Groups of data by patient populations

    d. Inappropriate optimization of payments by increasing length of stay

36. What is the basic formula for calculating each MS-DRG hospital payment?

    a. Hospital payment = MS-DRG relative weight × hospital base rate

    b. Hospital payment = MS-DRG relative weight × hospital base rate − 1

    c. Hospital payment = MS-DRG relative weight / hospital base rate + 1

    d. Hospital payment = MS-DRG relative weight / hospital base rate

37. What are the possible add-on payments that a hospital could receive in addition to the basic Medicare DRG payment?

    a. Additional payments may be made for locum tenens, increased emergency room services, stays over the average length of stay, and cost outlier cases.

    b. Additional payments may be made to critical access hospitals, for higher-than-normal volumes, unexpected hospital emergencies, and cost outlier cases.

    c. Additional payments may be made for increased emergency room services, critical access hospitals, increased labor costs, and cost outlier cases.

    d. Additional payments may be made to disproportionate share hospitals for indirect medical education, new technologies, and cost outlier cases.

38. What is the name of the national program to detect and correct improper payments in the Medicare fee-for-service (FFS) program?

    a. Medicare administrative contractors (MACs)

    b. Recovery audit contractors (RACs)

    c. Comprehensive error rate testing (CERT)

    d. Fiscal intermediaries (FIs)

39. The foundation of the CMS Hierarchical Condition Categories (HCCs) is _____ because they directly impact the risk score calculation

    a. ICD-10-CM diagnosis codes

    b. Denial and appeals

    c. HCPCS codes

    d. Quality audits

40. What is the database used by healthcare facilities to house billing information for all services provided to patients?

    a. Encoder

    b. Master patient index (MPI)

    c. Electronic health record (EHR)

    d. Chargemaster (CDM)

41. Which of the following situations would be identified by the NCCI edits?

    a. Determining the MS-DRG

    b. Billing for two services that are prohibited from being billed on the same day

    c. Whether data submitted electronically was successfully submitted

    d. Receiving the remittance advice

42. A hospital needs to know how much Medicare paid on a claim so they can bill the secondary insurance. What should the hospital refer to?

    a. Explanation of benefits

    b. Medicare Summary Notice

    c. Remittance advice

    d. Coordination of benefits

43. A patient has two health insurance policies: Medicare and a Medicare supplement. Which of the following statements is true?

    a. The patient receives any monies paid by the insurance companies over and above the charges.

    b. Monies paid to the healthcare provider cannot exceed charges.

    c. The decision on which company is primary is based on remittance advice.

    d. The patient should not have a Medicare supplement.

44. The purpose of a physician query is to _____.

    a. Identify the MS-DRG

    b. Identify the principal diagnosis

    c. Improve documentation for patient care and proper reimbursement

    d. Increase reimbursement as form of optimization

45. What is the term used when a Medicare hospital inpatient admission results in exceptionally high costs when compared to other cases in the same MS-DRG?

    a. Rate increase

    b. Charge outlier

    c. Cost outlier

    d. Budget surplus

46. What is the internet-only manual (IOM) published by CMS that provides a listing of all the topics included for Medicare coverage problems?

    a. Chargemaster (CDM)

    b. Medicare Learning Network (MLN)

    c. National Coverage Determination Manual (NCD)

    d. Regulatory Program Guide

47. A fee schedule is _____.

    a. Developed by third-party payers and includes a list of healthcare services, procedures, and charges associated with each

    b. Developed by providers and includes a list of healthcare services, procedures, and charges associated with each

    c. Developed by third-party payers and includes a list of healthcare services provided to a patient

    d. Developed by providers and lists charge codes

48. Which of the following general data elements does the charge description master *not* contain?

    a. Charge code description

    b. MS-DRG assignment

    c. Revenue code

    d. Price

49. If a provider believes a service may be denied by Medicare because it could be considered unnecessary, the provider must notify the patient before the treatment begins by using a(n) _____.

    a. Advance beneficiary notice (ABN)

    b. Advance notice of coverage (ANC)

    c. Notice of payment (NOP)

    d. Consent for payment (CFP)

50. Assignment of benefits is a contract between a physician and Medicare in which the physician agrees to bill Medicare directly for covered services and the beneficiary for the _____, and to accept the Medicare payment as payment in full.

    a. Coinsurance or deductible

    b. Deductible only

    c. Coinsurance only

    d. Balance of charges

51. A provision of the law that established the resource-based relative value scale (RBRVS) stipulates that refinements to relative value units (RVUs) must maintain _____.

    a. Moderate rate increases

    b. Market basket increases

    c. Budget neutrality

    d. Sustainable growth rate

52. The status indicator (SI) that identifies procedures, services, and supplies that are packaged into the cost and reimbursement for APC services with which they are most often performed is SI:

    a. A

    b. N

    c. F

    d. B

53. Identify the correct ICD-10-CM diagnosis code(s) and sequencing for a patient with disseminated candidiasis secondary to AIDS-related complex.

    a. B20, B37.7, Z20.6

    b. B37.7, B20

    c. B20, B37.7, Z21

    d. B20, B37.7

54. Identify the correct ICD-10-CM diagnosis code(s) and proper sequencing for urinary tract infection due to *E. coli.*

    a. N39.0

    b. N39.0, B96.20

    c. B96.20

    d. B96.20, N39.0

Domain 3 *Health Records and Data Content*

55. Which of the following includes names of the surgeon and assistants, date, duration, and description of the procedure and any specimens removed?

    a. Operative report

    b. Anesthesia report

    c. Pathology report

    d. Laboratory report

56. A patient with known COPD and hypertension under treatment was admitted to the hospital with symptoms of a lower abdominal pain. He undergoes a laparoscopic appendectomy and develops a fever. The patient was subsequently discharged from the hospital with a principal diagnosis of acute appendicitis and secondary diagnoses of postoperative infection, COPD, and hypertension. Which of the following diagnoses should *not* be tagged as present on admission (POA)?

    a. Postoperative infection

    b. Appendicitis

    c. COPD

    d. Hypertension

57. Which of the following would *not* be found in a medical history?

    a. Chief complaint

    b. Vital signs

    c. Present illness

    d. Review of systems

58. The overall goal of documentation standards is to ensure that _____.

    a. Physicians have access to the health record information they need to care for the patient

    b. The healthcare provider organization is reimbursed appropriately by payers

    c. The Centers for Medicare and Medicaid Services (CMS) do not find reason to fine the healthcare provider organization

    d. What is documented in the health record is complete and accurately reflects the treatment provided to the patient

59. The Joint Commission and CMS require hospitals to inform families of the opportunity to donate organs, tissue, or eyes. The name of the criteria that potential donors must meet is _____.

    a. United Network of Organ Sharing (UNOS)

    b. Conditions of Participation (CoP)

    c. Personal Health Record (PHR)

    d. Do Not Resuscitate (DNR)

60. What is the function of a consultation report?

    a. It provides a chronological summary of the patient's medical history and illness.

    b. It documents opinions about the patient's condition from the perspective of a physician not previously involved in the patient's care.

    c. It concisely summarizes the patient's treatment and stay in the hospital from the time of admission to the time of discharge.

    d. It documents the physician's instructions to other parties involved in providing care to a patient.

61. Which organization developed the first hospital standardization program?

    a. Joint Commission

    b. American Osteopathic Association

    c. American College of Surgeons

    d. American Association of Medical Colleges

62. The hospital is revising its policy on health record documentation. Currently, all entries in the health record must be legible, complete, dated, and signed. The committee chairperson wants to add that, in addition, all entries must have the time noted. However, another clinician suggests that adding the time of notation is difficult and rarely may be correct since personal watches and hospital clocks may not be coordinated. Another committee member agrees and says only electronic documentation needs a time stamp. Given this discussion, which of the following might the HIM director suggest?

    a. Note only hospital clock time in clinical documentation

    b. Only electronic documentation must have time noted

    c. Inform the committee that according to the Medicare Conditions of Participation, all documentation must be authenticated and dated

    d. Inform the committee that according to the Medicare Conditions of Participation, only medication orders must include date and time

63. When correcting erroneous information in a health record, which of the following is *not* appropriate?

    a. Print "error" above the entry

    b. Enter the correction in chronological sequence

    c. Add the reason for the change

    d. Use black pen to obliterate the entry

64. Which of the following is part of qualitative analysis review?

    a. Checking that only approved abbreviations are used

    b. Checking that all forms and reports are present

    c. Checking that documents have patient identification information

    d. Checking that reports that require authentication have signatures

65. External clinical validation audits are typically conducted on Medicare patients' health records by the:

    a. MACs

    b. RACs

    c. Medical staff reviewers

    d. Finance department staff

66. Who is responsible for writing and signing discharge summaries and discharge instructions?

    a. Attending physician

    b. Consulting physician

    c. Primary physician

    d. APRN

67. Where would a coder who needed to locate the histology of a tissue sample most likely find this information?

    a. Pathology report

    b. Progress notes

    c. Nurse's notes

    d. Operative report

68. A health information technician has been asked to design a problem list for an electronic health record (EHR). Which of the following data elements should be included on the problem list?

    a. Problem number, problem description, date problem entered

    b. Problem number, problem name, date of consent for treatment

    c. Patient identifying information, problem number, examination results

    d. Problem name, date of onset, physical exam

69. What data quality dimension is being jeopardized when a nurse uses the abbreviation CPR to mean cardiopulmonary resuscitation one time and computer-based patient record another time?

    a. Accuracy

    b. Consistency

    c. Precision

    d. Currency

70. An HIT, using her password, can access and change data in the hospital's master patient index. A billing clerk, using his password, cannot perform the same function. Limiting the class of information and functions that can be performed by these two employees is managed by _____.

    a. Network controls

    b. Password controls

    c. Administrative controls

    d. Access controls

Domain 4   *Compliance*

71. An HIM professional's ethical obligations _____.

    a. Apply regardless of employment site

    b. Are limited to the employer

    c. Apply to only the patient

    d. Are limited to the employer and patient

72. What should be done when the HIM department's error or accuracy rate is deemed unacceptable?

    a. A corrective action should be taken.

    b. The problem should be treated as an isolated incident.

    c. The formula for determining the rate may need to be adjusted.

    d. The problem area should be re-audited.

73. Statements that define the performance expectations and structures or processes that must be in place are _____.

    a. Rules

    b. Policies

    c. Guidelines

    d. Standards

74. A coding compliance program should contain the same components as the organization's:

    a. Quality improvement process

    b. Risk assessment plan

    c. Compliance plan

    d. Governing board policies

75. How are amendments handled in an EHR?

    a. Amendments are automatically appended to the original note; no additional signature is required.

    b. Amendments must be entered by the same person as the original note.

    c. Amendments cannot be entered more than 24 hours after the event's occurrence.

    d. The amendment must have a separate signature, date, and time.

76. Which of the following is *not* an accepted accrediting body for behavioral healthcare organizations?

    a. American Psychological Association

    b. Joint Commission

    c. Commission on Accreditation of Rehabilitation Facilities

    d. National Committee for Quality Assurance

77. What type of organization works under contract with CMS to conduct Medicare and Medicaid certification surveys for hospitals?

    a. Accreditation organizations

    b. Certification organizations

    c. State licensure agencies

    d. Conditions of participation agencies

78. The CDM captures charges for services including accommodations, room use, supplies, ancillary provisions and:

    a. Clinical services

    b. Insurance coverage

    c. Managed care

    d. Benefits

79. The component of the revenue cycle that is responsible for determining the appropriate financial class for the patient is:

    a. Submission of the claim

    b. Claims processing

    c. Claims reconciliation

    d. Pre-claims submission

80. Which of the following is a goal of the CDI program?

    a. Identify the providers who are not performing adequately

    b. Ensure that documentation is meeting the minimum standards for the medical staff bylaws

    c. Identify and clarify missing, conflicting, or nonspecific physician documentation related to diagnoses and procedures

    d. Alert hospital legal counsel concerning those physicians who are continually noncompliant

81. In a routine health record quantitative analysis review, it was found that a physician dictated a discharge summary on 1/26/20XX. The patient, however, was discharged two days later. In this case, what would be the best course of action?

    a. Request that the physician dictate another discharge summary.

    b. Have the record analyst note the date discrepancy.

    c. Request the physician dictate an addendum to the discharge summary.

    d. File the record as complete because the discharge summary includes all of the pertinent patient information.

82. Which of the following are the government inspectors whose mission is to reduce Medicare improper payments through the detection and collection of overpayments, identification of underpayments, and implementation of activities to prevent future improper payments?

    a. Health Care Fraud Prevention and Enforcement Team (HEAT)

    b. Medicare administration contractors (MACs)

    c. Medicare internal audit contractors (MICs)

    d. Recovery audit contractors (RACs)

Domain 5 | *Information Technologies*

83. A coding analyst consistently enters the wrong code for patient gender in the electronic billing system. What data quality or data integrity measures should be in place to ensure that only allowable code numbers are entered?

    a. Access controls

    b. Audit trail

    c. Edit checks

    d. Password controls

84. Which of the following would be the *best* technique to ensure that registration clerks consistently use the correct notation for assigning admission date in an electronic health record (EHR)?

    a. Make admission date a required field

    b. Provide an input mask for entering data in the field

    c. Make admission date a numeric field

    d. Provide sufficient space for input of data

85. CAC can help prevent fraudulent coding and ensure complete, consistent coding due to the:

    a. Complex coding

    b. NLP

    c. Efficiency of the encoder

    d. EHR format

86. A(n) _____ is computer software that assists in determining coding accuracy and reliability.

    a. Encoder

    b. Interface

    c. Diagnosis-related group

    d. Record locator service

87. The _____ uses expert or artificial intelligence software to automatically assign code numbers.

    a. Functional electronic health record (EHR)

    b. NHIN

    c. Natural language processing (NLP) encoding system

    d. Grouper

88. Which of the following is an example of a unique identifier for an individual health record to ensure that the information in the record is not misplaced, lost, or confused with information for another person each time a patient visits a facility?

    a. Account number

    b. Health record number

    c. Admission date

    d. Discharge date

89. The use of computer software that automatically generates a set of medical codes for review, validation, and use based on clinical documentation provided by healthcare practitioners is the definition of:

    a. Natural language processing

    b. Voice recognition

    c. Computer-assisted coding

    d. Electronic health record

90. The foundation of computer-assisted coding (CAC) that converts the human words into data that can be translated and manipulated by the computer system is:

    a. Encryption

    b. Natural language processing (NLP)

    c. Data algorithm administration

    d. Validation management

Domain 6   *Confidentiality and Privacy*

91. Which of the following is a threat to data security?

    a. Encryption

    b. People

    c. Red flags

    d. Access controls

92. Section 4004 of the 21st Century Cures Act identifies _____ exceptions that offer actors (namely, healthcare providers, health IT developers, HINs and HIEs) certainty that, when their practices access, exchange, or use health information that meet those conditions, the practice will not be considered information blocking.

    a. Zero

    b. Two

    c. Eight

    d. Ten

93. An employee in the physical therapy department arrives early every morning to snoop through the clinical information system for potential information about neighbors and friends. What security mechanisms should be implemented to prevent this security breach?

    a. Audit passwords

    b. Information access controls

    c. Facility access controls

    d. Workstation security

94. The method of encryption when two or more computers share the same secret key that is used to both encrypt and decrypt a message is called:

    a. Private key infrastructure

    b. Intrusion detection

    c. Digital screening

    d. Public key cryptography

95. Which of the following is the concept of the right of an individual to be left alone?

    a. Privacy

    b. Bioethics

    c. Security

    d. Confidentiality

96. Which of the following statements is true if a state law is stricter than HIPAA?

    a. HIPAA preempts state law.

    b. State law preempts HIPAA.

    c. A covered entity chooses which law to follow.

    d. The facility needs to consult an attorney.

97. Which of the following concepts limits disclosure of private matters including the responsibility to use, disclose, or release such information only with the knowledge and consent of the individual?

    a. Privacy

    b. Bioethics

    c. Security

    d. Confidentiality

98. Which of the following threatens the "need-to-know" principle?

    a. Backdating progress notes

    b. Blanket authorization

    c. HIPAA regulations

    d. Surgical consent

99. HealthSource is a business associate of Green Health System. A patient of Green Health System contacts HealthSource to request an accounting of disclosures, stating that this is his right per the HIPAA Privacy Rule. HealthSource:

    a. Does not need to respond to the patient because it is not a covered entity

    b. May refer the request to Green Health System

    c. Does not need to respond to the patient because this is not a HIPAA individual right

    d. Must respond to the patient and provide an accounting of disclosures

100. Every state has _____ that may include specific requirements for the content, format, retention and use of patient records.

    a. Licensure regulations

    b. Mandatory rules

    c. Clinical repositories

    d. Trauma registries

ANSWER KEY

CCA Practice Questions

1. **a** Index Carcinoma, in situ, see also Neoplasm, by site, in situ (Schraffenberger and Palkie 2022, 153).

2. **b** Index Melanoma (malignant), skin shoulder. Melanoma is considered a malignant neoplasm and is referenced as such in the index of ICD-10-CM. The term *benign neoplasm* is considered a growth that does not invade adjacent structures or spread to distant sites but may displace or exert pressure on adjacent structures (Schraffenberger and Palkie 2022, 157–159).

3. **b** CMS is responsible for updating the procedure classification (ICD-10-PCS) (Giannangelo 2019, 30).

4. **b** In ICD-10-CM, a condition that is produced by another illness or an injury and remains after the acute phase of the illness or injury is referred to as a sequela (Schraffenberger and Palkie 2022, 38).

5. **d** The seventh character provides information about encounter of care, such as initial encounter, subsequent encounter, or sequelae (Giannangelo 2019, 22–23).

6. **c** The fourth character captures etiology. The fifth captures anatomic site. The sixth captures severity (Giannangelo 2019, 22–23).

7. **a** Codes must be at least three characters, with a decimal point used after the third character (Giannangelo 2019, 22–23).

8. **b** When a note appears under a three-character code in ICD-10-CM, it applies to all codes within that category (Giannangelo 2019, 22–23).

9. **d** ICD-10-CM includes diagnoses only. In the development of the ICD-10 code sets, it was determined that creating a separate volume for procedures would be insufficient. Because of this, an entirely new procedure code system, ICD-10-PCS, was developed (Giannangelo 2019, 22–23).

10. **a** Coding Guideline I.A.12.a explicitly states this exception (CMS 2022a).

11. **a** Index Adenoma, adrenal (cortical). Index Syndrome, Conn's. According to the Index in ICD-10-CM, except where otherwise indicated, the morphological varieties of adenoma should be coded by site as for "Neoplasm, benign" (Schraffenberger and Palkie 2022, 152–153).

12. **a** CPT is a comprehensive descriptive listing of terms and codes for reporting diagnostic and therapeutic procedures and medical services (Giannangelo 2019, 56).

13. **c** Index Contusion, cerebral, right side. Add a sixth character of 1 for loss of consciousness of 30 minutes or less. Cerebral contusions are often caused by a blow to the head. A cerebral contusion is a more severe injury involving a bruise of the brain with bleeding into the brain tissue, but without disruption of the brain's continuity. The loss of consciousness that occurs often lasts longer than that of a concussion. Codes for cerebral laceration and contusion range from S06.31–S06.33 with sixth characters indicating whether a loss of consciousness or concussion occurred (Schraffenberger and Palkie 2022, 600–602).

14. d   The code selection is determined by measuring the greatest clinical diameter of the apparent lesion plus that margin required for complete excision (lesion diameter plus the most narrow margins required equals the excised diameter) (AMA 2021, 101).

15. c   Complex closure includes the repair of wounds requiring more than layered closure, namely, scar revision, debridement, extensive undermining, stents, or retention sutures (AMA 2021, 107).

16. a   Guideline I.C.15.q.2 Retained Products of Conception following an abortion: Subsequent admissions for retained products of conception following a spontaneous or legally induced abortion are assigned the appropriate code from category O03, spontaneous abortion, or codes O07.4, Failed attempted termination of pregnancy without complication and Z33.2, Encounter for elective termination of pregnancy. This advice is appropriate even when the patient was discharged previously with a discharge diagnosis of complete abortion (Schraffenberger and Palkie 2022, 509–510).

17. c   The term *urosepsis* is a nonspecific term and is not codable in ICD-10-CM. It is not to be considered synonymous with sepsis. It has no default code in the Alphabetic Index. Should a provider use this term, he or she must be queried for clarification (Schraffenberger and Palkie 2022, 122).

18. c   Guideline I.C.2.a: If treatment is directed at the malignancy, designate the malignancy as the principal diagnosis. The only exception to this guideline is if a patient admission or encounter is solely for the administration of chemotherapy, immunotherapy, or radiation therapy, assign the appropriate Z51.-code as the first-listed or principal diagnosis and the diagnosis or problem for which the service is being performed as a secondary diagnosis (Schraffenberger and Palkie 2022, 146–151).

19. b   Gastroenteritis is characterized by diarrhea, nausea, and vomiting, and abdominal cramps. Codes for symptoms, signs, and ill-defined conditions from Chapter 18 of the ICD-10-CM codebook are not to be used as the principal diagnosis when a related definitive diagnosis has been established. Patients can have several chronic conditions that coexist at the time of their hospital admission and qualify as additional diagnosis such as COPD and angina (Schraffenberger and Palkie 2022, 574–575).

20. c   In this circumstance, both codes F45.8 and G47.63 can be coded together because psychogenic dysmenorrhea is also an inclusion term; patient could have both conditions (CMS 2022a).

21. a   In the unusual instance when two or more diagnoses equally meet the criteria for principal diagnosis, as determined by the circumstances of admission, diagnostic workup, and the therapy provided, and the Alphabetic Index, Tabular List, or another coding guideline does not provide sequencing direction in such cases, any one of the diagnoses may be sequenced first (Schraffenberger and Palkie 2022, 96).

22. b   The APA developed the DSM to be the standard medical classification for mental disorders (Giannangelo 2019, 244).

23. c   A patient in status asthmaticus fails to respond to therapy administered during an asthmatic attack. This is a life-threatening condition that requires emergency care and likely hospitalization (Schraffenberger and Palkie 2022, 360).

24. d Signs, symptoms, abnormal test results, or other reasons for the outpatient visit are used when a physician qualifies a diagnostic statement as "rule out" or other similar terms indicating uncertainty. In the outpatient setting the condition qualified in that statement should not be coded as if it existed. Rather, the condition should be coded to the highest degree of certainty, such as the sign or symptom the patient exhibits. In this case, assign the code R07.9, Chest pain, unspecified (Schraffenberger and Palkie 2022, 105; Coding Guidelines Section IV.H.).

25. c For outpatient encounters for diagnostic tests that have been interpreted by a physician, and the final report is available at the time of coding, code any confirmed or definitive diagnosis(es) documented in the interpretation. Do not code related signs and symptoms as additional diagnosis. Note: This differs from the coding practice in the hospital inpatient setting regarding abnormal findings on test results (Schraffenberger and Palkie 2022, 104–105).

26. d O10.013, Pre-existing essential hypertension complicating pregnancy, third trimester. Z3A.30 is applicable to maternity patients aged 12–55 years inclusive (Schraffenberger and Palkie 2022, 520).

27. d CMS designed ICD-10-PCS with goals to improve coding accuracy, reduce training effort, and improve communication with physicians. It is not used to collect data about nursing care (Giannangelo 2019, 30–49).

28. c Additional signs and symptoms that may not be associated with a disease process should be coded when present (Schraffenberger and Palkie 2022, 36).

29. a Partial nephrectomy is an example of the root procedure Excision. A portion of the body part is cut out or off, without replacement (Giannangelo 2019, 36–40).

30. b The assignment of a diagnosis code is based on the provider's diagnostic statement that the condition exists (CMS 2022c, vi).

31. b Code I63.50 is assigned when the diagnosis states stroke, cerebrovascular, or cerebrovascular accident (CVA) without further specification. In this case, the patient had an occlusion without a stroke. Code I66.9 is assigned. The health record should be reviewed to make sure nothing more specific is available. Conditions resulting from an acute cerebrovascular disease, such as aphasia or hemiplegia, should be coded as well. The side that the hemiparesis is affecting is not stated, so code G81.90 is assigned (Schraffenberger and Palkie 2022, 329–331).

32. a Acute respiratory failure, code J96.00–J96.02, may be assigned as a principal or secondary diagnosis depending on the circumstances of the inpatient admission. Chapter-specific coding guidelines (obstetrics, poisoning, HIV, newborn) provide specific sequencing direction. Because the respiratory failure occurred after admission, it is listed as a secondary diagnosis and the congestive heart failure is listed first (Schraffenberger and Palkie 2022, 369–370).

33. d Guideline I.C.19.e.5(a): Adverse effects can occur in situations in which medication is administered properly and prescribed correctly in both therapeutic and diagnostic procedures. An adverse effect can occur when everything is done correctly. The first-listed diagnosis is the manifestation or the nature of the adverse effect, such as the hematuria. Locate the drug in the Substance column of the Table of Drugs and Chemicals in the Alphabetic Index to Diseases. Assign the appropriate seventh character to the drug or chemical code to identify whether the healthcare was provided during the initial encounter, a subsequent encounter, or for a sequela (Schraffenberger and Palkie 2022, 623–626).

34. c   Guideline I.C.9.e.1 for encounters occurring while the myocardial infarction is equal to, or less than, four weeks old, including transfers to another acute setting or a postacute setting, and the patient requires continued care for the myocardial infarction, codes from category I21 may continue to be reported (Schraffenberger and Palkie 2022, 319–320).

35. a   All claims involving inpatient admissions to general acute-care hospitals or other facilities that are subject to law or regulation mandating collection of present on admission information. Present on admission (POA) is defined as present at the time the order for inpatient admission occurs. Conditions that develop during an outpatient encounter, including emergency department, observation, or outpatient surgery, are considered POA. Any condition that occurs after admission is not considered a POA condition (Schraffenberger and Palkie 2022, 97).

36. b   Sepsis refers to a systemic immune response associated with the presence of pathological microorganisms or toxins in the blood, which can include bacteria, viruses, fungi, or other organisms. Code A41.01 is assigned for sepsis due to *Staphylococcus aureus*. Because abdominal pain is a symptom of diverticulitis, only the diverticulitis of the colon, unspecified part of colon, K57.92 is coded. Per Guideline I.C.1.d.4, if the reason for admission is both sepsis…and a localized infection…a code for the underlying systemic infection (sepsis) should be assigned first and the code for the localized infection (diverticulitis) should be assigned as a secondary diagnosis (Schraffenberger and Palkie 2022, 126–128).

37. c   Guideline I.C.2.d Primary malignancy previously excised is coded to category Z85, Personal history of malignancy neoplasm if there is no further treatment directed to that site and there is no evidence of any existing primary malignancy. Because the malignancy recurred, it is coded as a current malignancy, code C67.3, and no Z code is included (Schraffenberger and Palkie 2022, 148–149).

38. a   The physician or other qualified healthcare practitioner who is legally accountable for establishing the patient's diagnosis is acceptable because this information is typically documented by other clinicians involved in the patient's care (CMS 2022a, I.B.14).

39. d   Z codes are diagnosis codes and indicate a reason for healthcare encounter (Schraffenberger and Palkie 2022, 684).

40. d   Reposition S is the root operation. CG B3.1b CMS (Schraffenberger and Palkie 2022, 71).

41. d   Begin with the main term Repositioning; electrode, heart (Kuehn and Jorwic 2021, 101).

42. a   Medicare requires a Level II HCPCS code to identify a wound closed with tissue adhesives. Instead of assigning the CPT code for wound repair, G0168 should be assigned (Smith 2021, 84).

43. d   Modifier 24 is used for unrelated evaluation and management service by the same physician during a postoperative period (Smith 2021, 230).

44. d   One code is assigned for alcohol dependence with alcohol withdrawal. Alcohol abuse is not assigned per Excludes 1 note under F10.1. Under F10, the "use additional code" note for blood alcohol level (Y90.-) applies to this case since blood alcohol level is documented (Schraffenberger and Palkie 2022, 218–219).

45. **a** The anemia would be sequenced first based on principal diagnosis guidelines. Since the anemia is not specified as acute blood loss it's coded tochronic blood loss because "chronic" is a nonessential modifier for "blood loss anemia" (Schraffenberger and Palkie 2022, 93, 170–171).

46. **d** The patient was admitted for the senile cortical cataract and the procedures were completed for that condition. This follows the UHDDS guidelines for principal diagnosis selection. Per coding guidelines, there is an assumed causal relationship given between the type 2 diabetes and the cataract, so E11.36 would be correct (CMS 2022a).

47. **d** The patient was admitted, and COPD is listed as the principal diagnosis. Code J44.1 is used when the medical record includes documentation of COPD with acute exacerbation. ICD-10-CM presumes a cause-and-effect relationship and classifies chronic kidney disease with hypertension as hypertensive chronic kidney disease, code I12.9; however, the code also in category I12 directs the coding professional to also code the chronic renal failure N18.9 (Schraffenberger and Palkie 2022, 360).

48. **a** Code only confirmed cases. Confirmation does not require documentation of the type of test performed according to the Coding Guideline I.C.1.f (CMS 2022a).

49. **b** Repair of initial inguinal hernia, age six months to younger than five years old, with or without hydrocelectomy, reducible, is assigned 49500 (Smith 2021, 150–151).

50. **d** Modifiers are appended to the code to provide more information or to alert the payer that a payment change is required. Modifier 55 is used to indicate that the physician provided only postoperative care services for a particular procedure (Smith 2021, 53).

51. **b** Index main term: Destruction, hemorrhoid, thermal. Thermal includes infrared coagulation (Smith 2021, 149).

52. **c** These are multiple new problems that are presented with some risk (namely, trauma) and ordered two drugs, with management options evident (Smith 2021, 276).

53. **a** Index main term: Depression; then Index subterm: major, recurrent, *see* disorder, depressive, recurrent. The Index gives the following in the cross reference: Disorder, depressive, recurrent, current episode, severe (without mention of psychotic symptoms) F33.2 (Schraffenberger and Palkie 2022, 31–32).

54. **c** Main term for procedure: Excision; subterm: esophagus, upper (Schraffenberger and Palkie 2022, 59–62).

55. **d** Codes for symptoms, signs, and ill-defined conditions are not to be used as the principal diagnosis when a related definitive diagnosis has been established. The flank pain would not be coded because it is a symptom of the calculus. Root operation Dilation is coded because the intent is to expand the lumen of the tubular body part, the ureters. The stent is the device that is reported in the sixth character. One code is assigned for "bilateral" instead of two codes, indication "left, right" when a "bilateral" option is available (Schraffenberger and Palkie 2022, 35, 42).

56. **c** Main term for diagnosis: Incontinence; subterm: stress. Common procedural term: Suspension; subterm: urethra, *see* Reposition, Urinary System, table 0TS (Schraffenberger and Palkie 2022, 258, 614).

57. **c**   Index the main term of Hernia repair; inguinal; incarcerated. The age of the patient and the fact that the hernia is not recurrent makes 49507 the appropriate code (Smith 2021, 150–152).

58. **b**   Coding Guideline I.C.4.a.3 states that if the documentation identifies that the patient uses insulin but not the type of diabetes, the code assignment is E11 (CMS 2022a).

59. **b**   Main term of Hysteroscopy; lysis; adhesions (Smith 2021, 170).

60. **d**   In the abdomen, peritoneum, and omentum subsection, the exploratory laparotomy is a separate procedure and should not be reported when it is part of a larger procedure. The code of 49000 is not reported because laparotomy is the approach to the surgery. The code 58720 includes bilateral so modifier 50 is not necessary to report (Smith 2021, 170–172).

61. **c**   Dialysis, end-stage renal disease (ESRD). Code 90966 is for ESRD-related services for home dialysis per full month for patients 20 years and older (Smith 2021, 287).

62. **c**   Code 97113, Therapeutic procedure, one or more areas, each 15 minutes of aquatic therapy with therapeutic exercises, is billable per 15 minutes of therapy. The patient was treated for 30 minutes, so code 97113 should be reported twice. Modifier 50 is not applicable because the service is not a bilateral procedure (AMA 2021, 835).

63. **c**   In order to appropriately report administration of vaccines, both the product administered and the method of administration must be reported. An instructional note listed before CPT code 90476 states: "(For immune globulins, see codes 90281–90399. See codes 96365–96375 for administration of immune globulins)" (AMA 2021, 722–723).

64. **d**   Index Thyroidectomy, partial, resulting in code range 60210–60225 or Lobectomy, thyroid gland partial, resulting in code range 60210–60212. Review of the available codes indicates that code 60212 is correct because there is documentation of isthmusectomy and subtotal resection on the opposite (contralateral) side (AMA 2021, 454).

65. **b**   ICD-10-CM codes: O00.101

       ICD-10-CM rationale: The Alphabetic Index main term is Pregnancy, ectopic, tubal, right.

       ICD-10-PCS codes: 10T24ZZ

       ICD-10-PCS rationale: Per PCS Guideline C1: procedures performed on the products of conception are coded to the Obstetrics section. Procedures performed on the pregnant female other than the products of conception are coded to the appropriate root operation in the Medical and Surgical section.

       For code 10T24ZZ, the Alphabetic Index main term is Resection, subterm products of conception, ectopic. Reference Table 10T2 after Ectopic, then select Products of Conception for body part, select 4 Percutaneous endoscopic for the approach, select Z No Device for the device, and select Z No Qualifier for the qualifier (CMS 2022c, A.6).

66. **a**   The primary diagnosis code is benign prostatic hyperplasia (N40.1), which is found in the Alphabetic Index at the main term Hyperplasia, subterm prostate, with lower urinary tract symptoms. A use additional code note is present at N40.1 directing to assign additional codes for associated symptoms, so a secondary code is assigned for the urinary retention (R33.8). The Alphabetic Index main term is Retention, subterm urinary, specified. CPT code 53852 is accessed using Index Prostate, destruction, thermotherapy, radio frequency (Schraffenberger and Palkie 2022, 471–472; Smith 2021, 165).

67. **b**　When submitting a claim for a screening mammography and a diagnostic mammography for the same patient on the same day, attach modifier GG to the diagnostic mammography (AMA 2021, 923).

68. **a**　The geometric mean LOS (GMLOS) is defined as the total days of service, excluding any outliers or transfers, divided by the total number of patients (Casto and White 2021, 74).

69. **b**　Multiple surgical procedures with payment status indicator T performed during the same operative session are discounted. The highest-weighted procedure is fully reimbursed. All other procedures with payment status indicator T are reimbursed at 50 percent (Casto and White 2021, 108–110, 216–217).

70. **a**　There are not local coverage determinations (LCDs) and national coverage determinations (NCDs) for every type of procedure or service that could be provided for a patient (Casto and White 2021, 215–216).

71. **a**　Psychiatric and rehabilitation hospitals, long-term care hospitals, children's hospitals, cancer hospitals, and critical access hospitals are paid on the basis of reasonable cost, subject to payment limits per discharge or under a separate prospective payment system (PPS) (Miller 2020, 33–34).

72. **c**　Diagnosis-related groupings (DRGs) are classified by one of 25 major diagnostic categories (MDCs) (Casto and White 2021, 74–78).

73. **a**　Medicare Part A is generally provided free of charge to individuals age 65 and over who are eligible for Social Security. The coverage is provided to those with end-stage renal disease (Casto and White 2021, 35).

74. **b**　Critical access hospitals are paid on a cost-based payment system and are not part of the prospective payment system (Miller 2020, 34–35).

75. **a**　Third-party payers who reimburse providers on a fee-for-service basis generally update fee schedules on an annual basis (Casto and White 2021, 52–53).

76. **a**　Physicians submit claims via the electronic format (screen 837P), which takes the place of the CMS-1500 billing form (Casto and White 2021, 168–169).

77. **b**　To accept assignment means the provider or supplier accepts, as payment in full, the allowed charge based on the fee schedule (Casto and White 2021, 243).

78. **c**　Review the elements of the hospital compliance program with the employee (Foltz and Lankisch 2020, 511).

79. **b**　Since 1983, the prospective payment systems have been used to manage the costs of the Medicare and Medicaid programs (Casto and White 2021, 54–58).

80. **c**　Access to an indwelling IV or insertion of a subcutaneous catheter or port for the purpose of a therapeutic infusion is considered part of the procedure and not separately billed (Smith 2021, 302–303).

81. **a**　The goal of a compliance program is to reduce the liability with regards to fraud and abuse (Foltz and Lankisch 2020, 511–512).

82. **a**   Any secondary diagnoses assigned present on admission status will have a negative impact on reimbursement if no other code on the claim is assigned as a complication or comorbidity or a major complication or comorbidity (Brinda 2020, 184–185).

83. **c**   Payment for separately paid APCs depends on the status indicator assigned to each HCPCS code. This particular example allows separate payment on all five codes based on separately paid status indicator assignment (Casto and White 2021, 106–113).

84. **c**   Out-of-pocket expenses are the healthcare expenses that the insured party is responsible for paying after the insurer has paid its amount. In the example, after the allowed charges of 80 percent, or $400, are covered by the insurance company, the patient will be responsible for the remaining 20 percent, or $100 (Casto and White 2021, 15–25).

85. **a**   Managed fee-for-service (FFS) reimbursement is similar to traditional FFS reimbursement except that managed care plans control costs primarily by managing their members' use of healthcare services (Casto and White 2021, 25–32).

86. **d**   The case-mix index is 1.4500 for the total case-mix index of the hospital. An individual MS-DRG case mix can be figured by multiplying the relative weight of each MS-DRG by the number of discharges within that MS-DRG. This provides the total weight for each MS-DRG. The sum of all total weights (15,192) divided by the sum of total patient discharges (10,471) equals the case-mix index (Casto and White 2021, 227–232).

87. **d**   Discounting applies to multiple surgical procedures furnished during the same operative session. The full rate will be paid to the surgical procedure with the highest rate and the additional procedures will be discounted 50 percent of their APC rate (Casto and White 2021, 110, 126).

88. **b**   Medicare Part B, also known as supplemental medical insurance, covers physician and surgeon services and other Medicare-approved practitioners, ED and outpatient services, home health not covered under Part A, labs, x-rays, ASC services, physical and occupational therapies, and other services (Casto and White 2021, 35, 250).

89. **d**   Prior approval for a service or procedure is called precertification and allows coverage for a specific service (Casto and White 2021, 22–24).

90. **d**   Editing is not based on the clinical documentation of the discharge summary. Edits are predetermined based on coding conventions defined in the CPT codebooks, national and local policies and coding edits, analysis of standard medical and surgical practice, and review of current coding practices (Casto and White 2021, 217).

91. **a**   Portions of the NCCI are incorporated into the outpatient code editor (OCE) against which all ambulatory claims are reviewed. The OCE also applies a set of logical rules to determine whether various combinations of codes are correct and appropriately represent services provided (Smith 2021, 69–70).

92. **c**   Outpatient claims editor does not exist. Do not confuse this terminology with outpatient code editor (OCE) (Smith 2021, 236–237).

93. **b**   Clean claims are essential for accurate and timely reimbursement (Casto and White 2021, 169).

94. **a** Submitting paper claims subjects the claim to errors, whereas submitting electronic claims, using electronic health records, and auditing claims accuracy reduces the chance that the claim will contain inaccuracies or be incomplete (Casto and White 2021, 169).

95. **d** A procedure name is not a required element on a healthcare insurance claim (Casto and White 2021, 69–71).

96. **a** Value based purchasing (VBP) programs link quality to reimbursement (Casto and White 2021, 71).

97. **c** The pre-MDC assignment step was added to version 8, and identified a set of ICD-10-PCS procedures that crosses all major diagnostic categories (MDCs) (Casto and White 2021, 76).

98. **a** Some Medicare beneficiaries choose to participate in the Medicare Advantage plan, which provides expanded coverage of many healthcare services via different plans including HMOs, PPOs, private for-service plans, and special needs plans (Casto and White 2021, 35).

99. **c** Claims that automatically process through computer software are either auto-pay, auto-suspend, or auto-deny (Casto and White 2021, 168–169).

100. **b** Relative value units (RVUs) are assigned to each service to provide a value that correlates to payment (Casto and White 2021, 122–124).

101. **d** A service must not be solely for the convenience of the insured, the insured's family, or the provider (Casto and White 2021, 318–319).

102. **b** Coordination of benefits is necessary to determine which policy is primary and which is secondary so that there is no duplication of payments (Casto and White 2021, 24).

103. **b** A DRG is a predetermined amount of reimbursement for each Medicare inpatient (Casto and White 2021, 75).

104. **a** Physicians can prevent or minimize potentially abusive or fraudulent activities by developing a compliance plan (Casto and White 2021, 200–201).

105. **b** The case-mix index can be figured by multiplying the relative weight of each MS-DRG by the number of discharges within that MS-DRG (Casto and White 2021, 227–228).

106. **d** Eligibility standards for low income is a measure for Medicaid. Each state determines the standards according to federal guidelines (Casto and White 2021, 39–40).

107. **a** The Healthcare Common Procedural Coding System (HCPCS) identifies and groups the services within each APC group (Gordon 2020, 494).

108. **c** The Health Information Department along with both the Business Office and Cardiac Department should be consulted to determine where the breakdown of the charges and assignment of the procedure code occurs. Often one department assumes another department is submitting the code or charge and without auditing and communicating with each other on a regular basis, error can occur for long periods of time with either a financial gain or loss to the facility (Casto and White 2021, 208–215).

109. **a** HCPCS codes that are assigned in the charge description master that flow directly to the claim and bypass facility coding staff is a process known as hard coding (Casto and White 2021, 144–153).

110. **b** CMS implemented the CMS-HHCs in 2004 as a risk adjustment model, executed under the Medicare Advantage Program (Casto and White 2021, 59).

111. **b** The principal diagnosis determines the MDC assignment (Casto and White 2021, 74–76).

112. **b** A complication is a secondary condition that arises during hospitalization and is thought to increase the length of stay by at least one day for approximately 75 percent of the patients (Gordon 2020, 493).

113. **a** Results for lab tests will be included in a medical laboratory report (Brickner 2020a, 108).

114. **d** Results of an x-ray interpretation by a radiologist are reported in a radiography report (Brickner 2020a, 108).

115. **b** Pathological examinations of tissue samples and tissues or organs removed during surgical procedures are reported in the pathology report (Brickner 2020a, 108).

116. **a** Physician orders are the instructions a physician gives to the other healthcare professionals. Admission and discharge orders should be found for every patient (Brickner 2020a, 104–106).

117. **b** Benchmarking or peer comparison helps a manager to know how his or her team has performed compared to peers. This includes whether the case-mix index level puts the facility at risk (Casto and White 2021, 184).

118. **c** Clinical data document the patient's medical condition, diagnosis, and procedures performed as well as healthcare treatment provided (Brickner 2020a, 104).

119. **c** The operative report includes a description of the procedure performed (Brickner 2020a, 108).

120. **c** This information is collected by the examination of a newborn and reported on the newborn record (Sayles 2020, 85).

121. **c** An ECG is a report of an electrocardiogram of the heart (Brickner 2020a, 109).

122. **d** After an initial assessment, documentation by other allied health professionals varies by specialty with appropriate content and frequency of recording (Brickner 2020a, 103).

123. **c** Deidentified data in the health record are aggregated and turned into information that is used by public health professionals and researchers (Sayles 2020, 65).

124. **b** CMS requires health records to be maintained for at least five years (42 CFR 482.24(b); Johns 2020, 80)

125. **a** Subjective information includes symptoms and actions reported by the patient and not observed or measured by the healthcare provider (Reynolds 2020, 113, 121).

126. **b**   Objective information may be measured or observed by the healthcare provider (Reynolds 2020, 113, 121).

127. **d**   The plan includes orders and the roadmap for patient care (Reynolds 2020, 113, 121).

128. **c**   Professional conclusions reached from evaluation of the subjective or objective information make up the assessment (Reynolds 2020, 113, 121).

129. **a**   HIM professionals analyze health records for any missing reports, forms, or required signatures and deletions. This is a quantitative analysis of the health record (Reynolds 2020, 125–126).

130. **c**   Data integrity ensures that data is complete, accurate, and consistent (Brickner 2020b, 286).

131. **b**   Consistent data will be the same each time it is reported or collected (Sharp 2020, 199–204).

132. **a**   Clinical data document the patient's medical condition, diagnosis, and procedures performed as well as the healthcare treatment provided (Amatayakul 2020, 435–436).

133. **a**   Home health aides may assist the patient with activities of daily living such as bathing and housekeeping, which allows the patient to remain at home. Documentation of this type of intervention is also necessary (Reynolds 2020, 22–23, 120).

134. **c**   The emergency care record includes a pertinent history of the illness or injury and physical findings (Miller 2020, 41).

135. **d**   The pathology report includes descriptions of the tissue from a gross or macroscopic level and representative cells at the microscopic level (Brickner 2020a, 108).

136. **d**   The integrated health record is arranged so that the documentation from various sources is intermingled and follows strict chronological order (Brickner 2020a, 107, 116).

137. **b**   A complete medical history documents the patient's current complaints and symptoms and lists his or her past medical, personal, and family history (Brickner 2020a, 104).

138. **b**   The goal of a CDI program is to identify and clarify the missing, conflicting, or nonspecific physician documentation related to diagnoses and procedures (Brinda 2020, 188).

139. **b**   The consultation report documents the clinical opinion of a physician other than the primary or attending physician (Brickner 2020a, 109).

140. **c**   Physician orders are the instructions the physician gives to the other healthcare professionals (Brickner 2020a, 105–106).

141. **a**   Patient identity management relies on the master patient index (Sayles 2020, 70–72).

142. **d**   Medicare defines fraud as intentional deception or misrepresentation that results in an unauthorized benefit to an individual (Scott 2020, 118).

143. **c**   The OIG investigates and prosecutes individuals who overbill Medicare. It also develops an annual work plan that delineates the specific target areas that will be monitored in a given year (Casto and White 2021, 204).

144. **a** The disease index is a listing in diagnosis code number order for patients discharged from the facility during a particular time period. Each patient's diagnoses are converted from a verbal description to a numerical code, usually using a coding system such as ICD-10-CM (Brinda 2020, 163; Sayles and Gordon 2020, 731).

145. **d** Physician orders are the instructions the physician gives to the other healthcare professionals (Brickner 2020a, 105).

146. **b** The results of radiological and pathological procedures require interpretation by specially trained physicians called radiologists and pathologists. These physicians document their findings in written reports. The consultation report documents the clinical opinion of a physician other than the primary or attending physician (Brickner 2020a, 109).

147. **a** In a joint effort of the Department of Health and Human Services (HHS), Office of Inspector General (OIG), Centers for Medicare and Medicaid Services (CMS), and Administration on Aging (AOA), Operation Restore Trust was released in 1995 to target fraud and abuse among healthcare providers (Casto and White 2021, 201).

148. **d** Tracking length of stay is part of the hospital utilization review committee function (Casto and White 2021, 28–29).

149. **c** Refiling claims after a denial is not possible because denied claims must be appealed and is not a factor in controlling fraud and abuse (Casto and White 2021, 201–202).

150. **c** Any inappropriate payment made to a healthcare organization for any reason is considered an improper or inappropriate payment. Mistakes are errors. Other types of inappropriate payments are inefficiencies, abuse, and fraud (Casto and White 2021, 51, 252).

151. **c** Within the Coding Compliance Plan, using best practices to write a query to clarify documentation is a strategy to combat fraud and abuse in coding (Casto and White 2021, 192–196).

152. **d** Data reliability is a method of looking at data quality consistently. Reliability is frequently checked by having more than one person abstract data for the same case and compare the results for any discrepancies (Prater 2020, 622–623).

153. **c** The Health Insurance Portability and Accountability Act (HIPAA) of 1996 mandated incorporation of healthcare information standards into all electronic or computer-based health information systems (Miller 2020, 56).

154. **a** HL7 developed the HL7 Electronic Health Record System (EHR-S) Functional Model. It also includes many standards for data exchange with patient information (Brinda 2020, 174).

155. **a** The privacy officer must report any breaches of secured data to the Office of Civil Rights (OCR) via the Department of Health and Human Services (HHS) (Rinehart-Thompson 2020b, 271).

156. **b** A valid authorization must include a description of the information to be used or disclosed, a statement concerning redisclosure, and the expiration date (Rinehart-Thompson 2020b, 281).

157. **b** An audit trail is a record of all transactions in the computer system, which is maintained and reviewed for instances of unauthorized access (Sayles 2020, 81).

158. **c**   The False Claims Act was passed during the Civil War. The law is the foundation upon which fraud and abuse efforts have been based (Brickner 2020a, 118).

159. **c**   Performance counseling usually begins with informal counseling or a verbal warning. No record is kept in the employee's file (Leblanc 2020, 710–712).

160. **b**   Establish a process, such as a hotline, to receive complaints and adopt procedures to protect the anonymity of complainants and to protect whistleblowers from retaliation (O'Dell 2020, 616–617).

161. **d**   All newly hired coding personnel should receive extensive training on the facility's and HIM department's compliance programs. Education of the medical staff on documentation is likewise important to the success of any compliance program (Palkie 2020, 301–308).

162. **d**   The OIG has issued compliance program guidance since 1998 (Palkie 2020, 301–302).

163. **c**   Upcoding is the practice of assigning a diagnosis or procedure code specifically for the purpose of obtaining a higher level of payment (Hunt and Kirk 2020, 296).

164. **b**   The CDM coordinator will need to plan for the review of the CMS system payment rules and the incorporation of the rule changes into the CDM (Casto and White, 2021, 152).

165. **d**   A joint effort of the HHS and the DOJ, the mission of the Health Care Fraud Prevention Team (HEAT) is to prevent waste, fraud and abuse, reduce healthcare costs, improve quality of care for Medicare and Medicaid patients, and provide best practice information (Palkie 2020, 307–308).

166. **d**   Two types of queries used in clinical documentation integrity (CDI) are paper and electronic (Brinda 2020, 188).

167. **c**   Fraud is an intentional representation that an individual knows to be false or does not believe to be true and knowingly misrepresents the act, which could result in an unauthorized benefit (Casto and White 2021, 200).

168. **d**   The cornerstone of accurate coding is physician documentation. Ensuring the accuracy of coded data is a shared responsibility between the coding professional and physicians (Brinda 2020, 183–188).

169. **b**   Because of the risks associated with miscommunication, verbal orders are discouraged. When a verbal order is necessary, a clinician should sign, give his or her credential (for example, RN, PT, or LPN), and record the date and time the order was received. Verbal orders for medication are usually required to be given to, and to be accepted only by, nursing or pharmacy personnel (Brickner 2020a, 106).

170. **c**   Recovery audit contractors (RACs) would become a cost-effective means of ensuring correct payments to providers under Medicare. The RACs were charged with identifying underpayments and overpayments for claims filed under Medicare (Foltz and Lankisch 2020, 506).

171. **b**   An input mask shows the format in which data will be displayed in the EHR (Sayles 2020, 83).

172. **c**   The type of tool used to aid in the coding process is called an encoder (Sayles 2020, 87).

173. **b**   Some healthcare organizations are now using computer-assisted coding (CAC), which uses EHR data to assign the codes (Sayles 2020, 87).

174. **b**   Natural language processing (NLP) is an artificial intelligence software that reads digital text from online documents and suggests codes to match the documentation (Sayles 2020, 82).

175. **b**   Some encoders are built using expert system techniques such as rule-based systems, and other encoding software is more simplistic, merely automating a look-up function similar to the manual index in ICD or other coding classifications (Sayles 2020, 87).

176. **a**   Communications and network technologies—used by providers to enter orders for medications, lab tests, and other services—are the computerized provider order entry system (CPOE) (Amatayakul 2020, 324).

177. **b**   One potential area for poor data quality surrounds the need for making data entry easier. These include copy and paste, macros, standard orders, and other techniques that reuse data. These techniques can make data entry faster, but care must be taken to ensure appropriate modification to the specific patient (Brickner 2020a, 105).

178. **c**   A clinical decision support system delivers targeted clinical decision support by supplying clinical reminders and alerts (Bowe and Williamson 2020, 370).

179. **b**   Concurrent review occurs on a continuing basis during a patient's stay (Reynolds 2020, 126).

180. **b**   Data integrity means that the values are consistent throughout the hospital information systems (Brickner 2020b, 314).

181. **b**   Confidentiality is a legal ethical concept that establishes the healthcare provider's responsibility for protecting health records and other personal and private information from unauthorized use or disclosure (Rinehart-Thompson 2020b, 248).

182. **b**   By creating a Durable Power of Attorney for Healthcare Decisions (DPOA-HCD), an individual, while still competent, designates another person (proxy) to make healthcare decisions consistent with the individual's wishes on his or her behalf (Rinehart-Thompson 2020a, 231).

183. **b**   A subpoena is a direct command that requires an individual or a representative of an organization to appear in court or to present an object to the court (Rinehart-Thompson 2020a, 227).

184. **b**   The Privacy Rule introduced the standard of minimum necessary to limit the amount of PHI used, disclosed, and requested. This means that healthcare providers and other covered entities must limit uses, disclosures, and requests to only the amount needed to accomplish the intended purpose (Rinehart-Thompson 2020b, 249).

185. **a**   It is generally agreed that social security numbers (SSNs) should not be used as patient identifiers (Sayles 2020, 83–84).

186. **c**   The Notice of Privacy Practices includes a statement that the covered entity reserves the right to change the terms of its notice and to make the new notice provisions effective for all PHI that it maintains (Rinehart-Thompson 2020b, 249).

187. **a**   The 21st Century Care Act, Section 4004 was instituted to define the practices of information blocking; it also authorized the Secretary of HHS to identify those activities that do not constitute information blocking, or "exceptions" (AHIMA 2020).

188. **d**   The Information Governance Principles for Healthcare (IGPHC) includes the Principle of Retention that states, "An organization shall maintain its information for an appropriate time, taking into account its legal, regulatory, fiscal, operational, risk, and historical requirements" (Johns 2020, 80).

189. **c**   Encryption is the process of transforming text into an unintelligible string of characters that can be transmitted via communications media with a high degree of security and then decrypted when it reaches a secure destination (Brickner 2020b, 302).

190. **d**   The HIPAA Privacy Rule regarding fundraising states that individuals must be informed if their information is used for fundraising purposes (Rinehart-Thompson 2020b, 280).

191. **c**   Covered entities must retain policies for six years from the date of creation or when it was last in effect (Rinehart-Thompson 2020b, 250).

192. **c**   The Notice of Privacy Practices must be given to every patient the first time they come to the facility for care (Rinehart-Thompson 2020b, 260).

193. **a**   A clinical data repository is a database structure that supports an extensive number of data entries and retrievals, differentiated from a clinical data warehouse that performs analytics on data in its database (Amatayakul 2020, 340).

194. **d**   A portal is a special application to provide secure remote access to specific applications (Amatayakul 2020, 325).

195. **d**   The Office of the National Coordinator (ONC) developed the vision and mission with direction from the federal government's Federal Health IT Strategic Plan 2015–2020 (Sayles 2020, 249–250).

196. **a**   Data definition means that the data and information documented in the health record are defined; users of the data must understand what the data mean and represent (Brinda 2020, 179).

197. **a**   The terminal digit filing system is considered the most efficient because it evenly distributes health records throughout the filing units (Sayles 2020, 73).

198. **b**   Electronic signature authentication systems require the author to sign into the system with a user ID and password, review the document to be signed, and indicate approval (Brickner 2020a, 127).

199. **d**   In both the MS-DRG and APC groupings, coding professionals enter the codes that have been selected in a computer program called a grouper. The grouper then assigns the patient's case to the correct group based on the ICD-10-CM or CPT/HCPCS codes (Sayles 2020, 87).

200. **b**   Computer viruses and other malware constitute a threat to data security (Brickner 2020b, 291).

1. **d** Index Fracture, traumatic, femur, capital epiphyseal. Seventh character is required for further classification of an episode of care and the healing status (Schraffenberger and Palkie 2022, 587–588).

2. **d** Index either Neonatal, tooth, teeth K00.6, or Eruption, teeth/tooth (Schraffenberger and Palkie 2022, 385–386).

3. **a** CPT code 21012 describes excision of a subcutaneous soft tissue tumor of the face or scalp greater than 2 cm and is appropriately coded when the tumor is removed from the subcutaneous tissue rather than subgaleal or intramuscular. Simple and intermediate closure of the wound is included in the procedure for the excision in the musculoskeletal section of CPT (AMA 2021, 150).

4. **c** Code 19125 describes an excision of a lesion that was identified by preoperative placement of a radiological marker (AMA 2021, 125).

5. **d** Open skull fracture: The Alphabetic Index main term is Fracture, traumatic. The specific site of the skull fracture is not stated within the diagnostic statement. The seventh character B is assigned to indicate the fracture is open and this is the initial encounter. Subarachnoid hemorrhage: The Alphabetic Index main term is Hemorrhage with subterms intracranial, subarachnoid, traumatic. Subdural hemorrhage: The Alphabetic Index main term is Injury with subterms intracranial, subdural hemorrhage (traumatic). For the subdural and subarachnoid hemorrhage code assignments, the sixth character 7 is selected upon review of the Tabular List to indicate the loss of consciousness with death due to brain injury, prior to regaining consciousness and the seventh character A is assigned to represent the initial encounter (Schraffenberger and Palkie 2022, 593–594).

6. **d** ICD-10-PCS classifies cardiac pacemakers as Devices, character 6. Root operations of Insertion, removal, and revision always involve a device, such as a pacemaker. In coding initial insertion of a dual chamber permanent pacemaker, three codes are required—one for the pacemaker (0JH606Z) and one for each lead (02H63JZ, 02HK3JZ) (Schraffenberger and Palkie 2022, 340–341).

7. **c** Extirpation is the root operation for taking or cutting out solid material from a body part. For a thrombectomy, the thrombus is the solid material removed. The Alphabetic Index main term is Thrombectomy, *see* Extirpation. Following the cross-reference, the main term is Extirpation, Vein, Cephalic, Right 05CD. Reference the 05C table for the remaining characters of the code. The body part value is the right cephalic vein (D), the approach is open (0), and there is no device or qualifier (Z), resulting in code 05CD0ZZ (Kuehn and Jorwic 2021, 87–89).

8. **b** ICD-10-CM classifies both Mobitz type I and type II to I44.1 (Schraffenberger and Palkie 2022, 327–328).

9. **a** Index Checking (of), cardiac pacemaker, pulse generator, Z45.010. The pacemaker check is the root operation Measurement. Index: Measurement, Cardiac, Pacemaker 4B02XSZ (Schraffenberger and Palkie 2022, 340–342).

10. c   Coding Guideline I.C.9.a.2 states to assign codes from category I12, when both hypertension and a condition classifiable to category N18, Chronic kidney disease (CKD), are present (CMS 2022a).

11. c   Index Bypass, Artery, Coronary, One artery. One artery is selected since there two different qualifiers (character 7). One qualifier is "8 Internal Mammary, Right," and the other is "9 Internal Mammary, Left." Internal mammary-coronary artery bypass is accomplished by loosening the internal mammary artery from its normal position and using the internal mammary artery to bring blood from the subclavian artery to the occluded coronary artery. Codes are selected based on whether one or both internal mammary arteries are used (Schraffenberger and Palkie 2022, 338–339).

12. c   The Judkins technique provides x-ray imaging of the coronary arteries by introducing one catheter into the femoral artery with maneuvering up into the left coronary artery orifice, followed by a second catheter guided up into the right coronary artery, and subsequent injection of a contrast material (Schraffenberger and Palkie 2022, 338–339).

13. a   Z51.81, Encounter for, Therapeutic drug monitoring, is the correct code to use when a patient visit is for the sole purpose of undergoing a laboratory test to measure the drug level in the patient's blood or urine or to measure a specific function to assess the effectiveness of the drug. Z51.81 may be used alone if the monitoring is for a drug that the patient is on for only a brief period, not long term. However, there is a "code also" note under this code to remind the coding professional to code for any associated long-term current drug use with codes from category Z79 (Schraffenberger and Palkie 2022, 704).

14. b   Endoscopy, colon, exploration; procedure was not completed (AMA 2021, 380, 1092).

15. c   Code 43761 describes the repositioning of the nasogastric tube. If imaging guidance is performed, assign 76000 (AMA 2021, 365).

16. b   Index Abortion, threatened (spontaneous) O20.0. Hemorrhage is included in the code per the Includes notes under O20.0. Category Z3A, Weeks of gestation, is assigned as an additional code for all pregnancy and childbirth codes per the "use additional code" note at the beginning of Chapter 15 (Schraffenberger and Palkie 2022, 511–512).

17. b   Index Rash, diaper, L22 (Schraffenberger and Palkie 2022, 414–415).

18. c   Coding Guideline I.C.12.a.5 notes that pressure ulcers present on admission but healed at the time of discharge are assigned the code for site and stage at time of admission (CMS 2022c).

19. b   The Alphabetic Index main term is Shock with subterm anaphylactic, due to food, nuts. The seventh character A is used for the initial encounter (CMS 2022a, 1172).

20. d   Osteomyelitis, infection of bone, is subdivided into fourth-digit subcategories and fifth and sixth character subclassifications for laterality. Use additional code for infectious agent (Schraffenberger and Palkie 2022, 452).

21. b   Code 99204 meets two of the three required elements for the medical decision-making (Smith 2021, 257).

22. **b**   Index Anemia, aplastic, due to, drugs, D61.1. A coding professional should always assign the most specific type of anemia. Anemia due to chemotherapy is often aplastic. There is a "use additional code for adverse effect" note at D61.1 to assign an additional code to identify the drug causing the anemia. Utilize the Table of Drugs and Chemicals to locate the term Antineoplastic NEC. Then follow the row across to the Adverse effect column to locate the code. A seventh character of D is used to indicate "subsequent encounter" (Schraffenberger and Palkie 2022, 148).

23. **c**   Index Examination, well baby, Z00.129, for the routine well-child examination. Index, Premature, infant—*see* Preterm, newborn, unspecified weeks of gestation. P07.30 is assigned as an additional code per Guideline I.C.16.e (Schraffenberger and Palkie 2022, 684).

24. **c**   Certain signs and symptoms of breast disease are included in category N64, Other disorders of breast, which are in Chapter 14: Diseases of the genitourinary system (Schraffenberger and Palkie 2022, 475).

25. **b**   Devices used as part of the procedure and removed as the procedure concludes are not assigned the ICD-10-PCS sixth character (Kuehn and Jorwic 2021, 19)

26. **a**   Per Coding Guideline I.C.12.a.6, if a patient is admitted with a pressure ulcer at one stage and it progresses to a higher stage, two separate codes should be assigned—one code for the site and stage on admission and a second code for the same site at the highest stage (CMS 2022c).

27. **d**   Index Cholecystectomy, *see* Resection, Gallbladder, table 0FT4 because the whole gallbladder was removed. The laparoscopy is the approach and is not coded separately per 2014 ICD-10-PCS Official Guidelines for Coding and Reporting, Guideline B3.11a (page 8) "Inspection of a body part performed in order to achieve the objective of a procedure is not coded separately." To build the code, locate table 0FT and body part 4 Gallbladder, then 4 Percutaneous Endoscopic for the approach, then Z No device for device, and Z No qualifier for the qualifier (Schraffenberger and Palkie 2022, 399–401).

28. **b**   The physician or hospital will report 32554 for the first thoracentesis and 32554-76 with modifier 76, Repeat procedure or service by same physician (Smith 2021, 56).

29. **b**   *CPT Assistant* provides additional CPT coding guidance on how to assign a CPT code by providing intent on the use of the code and explanation of parenthetical instructions. The American Medical Association publishes the guidance monthly (AMA 2021, xix).

30. **a**   ICD-10-CM Alphabetic Index Osteoarthritis, primary, laterality for left hip M16.1-. ICD-10-PCS Index keyword is Replacement, joint, hip 0SRB (Schraffenberger and Palkie 2022, 436–437).

31. **b**   An encoder is a computer software program designed to assist coding professionals in assigning appropriate clinical codes and to help ensure accurate reporting of diagnoses and procedures (Sayles 2020, 75).

32. **c**   Medicare revamped the DRG system to incorporate severity of illness into the MS-DRG payment system in fiscal year 2008 (Casto and White 2021, 75).

33. **c**   Tricare is the healthcare program for active duty members of the military and other qualified family members (Casto and White 2020, 43–44).

34. b Unbundling occurs when a panel code exists, and the individual tests are reported rather than the panel code (Smith 2021, 69, 199).

35. a Reporting additional test codes that overlap codes in a panel allows the coding professional to assign all appropriate codes for services provided. It is inappropriate to assign additional panel codes when all codes in the panel are not performed. Reporting individual lab codes is appropriate when all codes in a panel have not been provided (Smith 2021, 214–215).

36. a The OIG's Compliance Program Guidance for Hospitals recommends that hospitals appoint a chief compliance officer and establish a compliance committee to provide assistance (Casto and White 2021, 189–192).

37. b The front end of the revenue cycle management process includes scheduling and registration, insurance verification, preauthorization, financial counseling and pre-encounter services. Claims appeals are a back-end process (Casto and White 2021, 233–264).

38. c AHA's *Coding Clinic for ICD-10-CM/PCS* is a quarterly publication of the Central Office on ICD-10-CM/PCS, which allows coding professionals to submit a request for coding advice through the coding publication. AHA's *Coding Clinic* is the only official publication for ICD-10-CM and ICD-10-PCS coding guidelines and advice provided by the four Cooperating Parties (Smith 2021, 8, 41).

39. b CMS developed MUEs to prevent providers from billing units in excess and receiving inappropriate payments. This new editing was the result of the outpatient prospective payment system that pays providers based on the HCPCS/CPT code and units. Payment is directly related to units for specified HCPCS/CPT codes assigned to an ambulatory payment classification (CMS 2022a, I-5–I-6).

40. c The documentation of the charges and itemized bill is not the responsibility of the physician (Smith 2021, 9–10).

41. d The identity of the patient's nearest relative and an emergency contact number are not relative to securing payment from the insurer. The encounter should include the date of the encounter and the identity of the observer (Smith 2021, 9–10).

42. b The hospital will receive the same reimbursement regardless of the length of stay (Casto and White 2021 51–65).

43. c Home health resource groups (HHRGs) represent the classification system established for the prospective reimbursement of covered home care services to Medicare beneficiaries during a 60-day episode of care (Casto and White 2021, 154).

44. c One section of the Affordable Care Act established the Hospital Readmissions Reduction Program, requiring CMS to reduce payments to the IPPS hospitals for discharges beginning October 1, 2012 (Casto and White 2021, 58, 60).

45. b The CMS-HCC model is used to create a risk score for each beneficiary (Casto and White 2021, 60).

46. a Children's hospitals are excluded from the Medicare acute-care PPS because the PPS diagnosis-related groups do not accurately account for the resource costs for the types of patients treated (Hazelwood 2020, 230–240).

47. **c** CMS identified hospital-acquired conditions (not present on admission) as "reasonably preventable," and hospitals do not receive additional payment for cases in which these conditions are not present on admission (Hazelwood 2020, 231).

48. **c** Gram-negative pneumonia is not on CMS's list of diagnoses that are considered to be hospital-acquired conditions (HACs). HACs (not present on admission) are considered to be "reasonably preventable," and hospitals do not receive additional payment for cases in which one of the conditions was not present on admission (Hazelwood 2020, 230–231).

49. **c** The focus on the delivery, measurement, and provision of quality patient care led to value-based purchasing initiatives, which include POA, HACs, and SREs (Casto and White 2021, 71, 256).

50. **d** The number of APCs reportable per encounter is unlimited (Casto and White 2021, 170).

51. **a** Each code in the HCPCS has been assigned a payment status indicator that establishes how a service, procedure or item is paid in OPPS (Casto and White 2021, 109).

52. **c** Addendums should be dated the day that the addendum was created (Brickner 2020a, 78).

53. **d** The seven characteristics of high-quality documentation include clarity, completeness, consistency, legibility, preciseness, reliability, and timeliness (Casto and White 2022, 193).

54. **a** Auto-authentication is a policy that allows the physician or provider to state in advance that dictated and transcribed reports should automatically be considered approved and signed when the physician does not make corrections within a certain period of time. Another variation of auto-authentication is that physicians authorize the HIM department to send a weekly list of documents needing signatures. The list is then signed and returned to the HIM department (Brickner 2020a, 103).

55. **b** Among the concerns with healthcare operations and development of bylaws is ensuring that the information documented in the patient record supports patient care as well as quality improvement activities and accreditation (Sharp 2020, 189).

56. **a** The discharge summary provides an overview of the entire medical encounter to ensure the continuity of future care by providing information to the patient's attending physician, referring physician, and any consulting physicians; to provide information to support the activities of the medical staff review committee; and to provide concise information that can be used to answer information requests from authorized individuals or entities (Brickner 2020a, 109).

57. **b** Under HIPAA, at the time of admission or prior to treatment, patients must be informed about the use of individually identifiable health information. The Notice of Privacy Practices is signed by the patient (Rinehart-Thompson 2020b, 262).

58. **c** The chief complaint is the nature and duration of the symptoms that caused the patient to seek medical attention as stated in the patient's own words (Brickner 2020a, 104).

59. **a** Clinical information is data related to the patient's diagnosis or treatment in a healthcare facility (Brickner 2020a, 104).

60. **d** Financial data include details about the patient's occupation, employer, and insurance coverage (Brickner 2020a, 103–104).

61. **b** Three types of matching algorithms are found in the MPI. These are the deterministic algorithm, the probabilistic algorithm, and the rules-based algorithm. The rules-based assigns weights to specific data elements and uses the weights to compare one record to another (Sayles 2020, 72).

62. **b** In the MPI, an overlay occurs when a patient is erroneously assigned another person's health record number (Sayles 2020, 72).

63. **a** The transfer or referral form provides document communication among caregivers in multiple healthcare settings. It is important that a patient's treatment plan be consistent as the patient moves through the healthcare delivery system (Brickner 2020a, 110).

64. **c** According to the Joint Commission, except in emergency situations, every surgical patient's chart must include a report of a complete history and physical conducted no more than seven days before the surgery is to be performed (Brickner 2020a, 99–100).

65. **a** According to Medicare Conditions of Participation, the physical examination must be completed within 24 hours of admission (Brickner 2020a, 97, 112).

66. **b** An incomplete record not rectified within a specific number of days as indicated in the medical staff rules and regulations is considered to be delinquent (Johns 2020, 76–77).

67. **d** Retrospective reviews occur after the patient is discharged (Johns 2020, 77).

68. **b** The benefit of concurrent review is that content or authentication issues can be identified at the time of patient care and rectified in a timely manner (Johns 2020, 76–77, 416).

69. **c** The HIM manager may compare organizational data with external data from peer groups to determine best practices (Prater 2020, 621–622).

70. **a** Quantitative analysis looks for the presence of documents and signatures (Brickner 2020a, 76–77).

71. **d** Surveyors review the documentation of patient care services to determine whether the standards for care are being met (Brickner 2020a, 82–87).

72. **c** Participating organizations must follow the Medicare Conditions of Participation to receive federal funds from the Medicare program for services rendered (Brickner 2020a, 97, 112).

73. **b** Every healthcare facility should have a compliance program—a set of internal policies and procedures that are put into place to comply with federal and state laws (Palkie 2020, 301–306).

74. **c** The Physician Self-Referral Law, known as the Stark Law, builds on the Anti-Kickback Statute and prohibits a physician from referring patients to a business in which he or she is a member (Foltz and Lankisch 2020, 504).

75. **c** Seven elements are required as part of the basic elements of a corporate compliance program. A medical staff appointee is not one of these required elements (Palkie 2020, 301–306).

76. **d** Quality improvement (QI) programs have been in place in hospitals for years and have been required by the Medicare or Medicaid programs and accreditation standards. QI programs have covered medical staff as well as nursing and other departments or processes (Miller 2020, 27–28).

77. **a** The coding professional is not following Standard 6 of AHIMA Standards of Ethical Coding, which states that all healthcare data elements required for external reporting purposes, including quality and patient safety measurements, are to be reported (Hamilton 2020, 671–672).

78. **a** Two types of physician queries are open-ended and multiple-choice queries (Brinda 2020, 187).

79. **b** Maintenance of the CDM requires expertise in coding, clinical procedures, health record or clinical documentation, and billing regulations (Handlon 2020, 258).

80. **a** CDM software is primarily designed to continuously apply edits to point out compliance issues, check validity of CPT and revenue codes, and identify items priced below national reimbursement levels (Handlon 2020, 258).

81. **c** Vocabulary standards establish common definitions for medical terms to encourage consistent descriptions of an individual's condition in the health record (Giannangelo 2019, 434).

82. **a** The basic inpatient CDI process can be divided into three main functions: record review, query for documentation clarification and physician education (Casto and White 2021, 192).

83. **a** The AHIMA Standard of Ethical Coding sets forth guidelines that all coding and billing professionals understand in ethical decision making (Hamilton 2020, 671–672).

84. **d** Interoperability is the capability of two or more information systems and software applications to communicate and exchange information (Brinda 2020, 174).

85. **a** Encoders come in two distinct categories: logic-based and automated codebook formats. A logic-based encoder prompts the user through a variety of questions and choices based on the clinical terminology entered. The coding professional selects the most accurate code for a service or condition (and any possible complications or comorbidities). An automated codebook provides screen views that resemble the actual format of the coding system (Sayles 2020, 87).

86. **d** Electronic data interchange allows the transfer (incoming and outgoing) of information directly from one computer to another by using standard formats (Amatayakul 2020, 348, 382–384).

87. **a** Unstructured data are data that do not have a predefined data model or are not stored in a traditional database structure. Unstructured data are typically found in documents, emails, and images (Johns 2020, 83–84).

88. **c** While CAC is used mainly for the coding of the health record for reimbursement purposes, another purpose is the automation of CDI (Brinda 2020, 185).

89. **b** The ability to immediately edit is the benefit of front-end speech recognition (Sayles 2020, 82).

90. **b** The definition of semantic is "meaning." In order to have a common meaning across disparate systems there must be a standard vocabulary to impart such meaning (Amatayakul 2020, 340).

91. **b** A valid authorization includes an expiration date or event. The authorization has to have enough information to identify the patient (Rinehart-Thompson 2020a, 227).

92. **c** Methods of authentication include smart cards, biometrics and passwords (Brickner 2020b, 298).

93. b Privacy is the right of an individual to be left alone. It includes freedom from observation or intrusion into one's private affairs and the right to maintain control over certain personal and health information (Rinehart-Thompson 2020b, 248, 265).

94. a The Final Rule that defines practices which constitute information blocking and authorizes the Secretary of Health and Human Services (HHS) to identify reasonable and necessary activities that do not constitute information blocking (referred to as "exceptions") is the Cures Act (HealthIT.gov 2022).

95. c Notice of Privacy Practices must be given to all patients the first time they come to the facility for care (Rinehart-Thompson 2020b, 260).

96. c The OIG believes that compliance programs will benefit by identifying and preventing criminal and unethical conduct, in addition to the other benefits listed (Brickner 2020b, 302).

97. c Destruction of records factors are applicable federal and state statutes and regulations, accreditation standards, pending or ongoing litigation, storage capabilities and cost (Rinehart-Thompson 2020a, 238).

98. a Audit trails can provide tracking information such as who accessed which records and for what purpose (Sayles 2020, 81, 88).

99. a Role-based access control (RBAC) is a control system in which access decisions are based on the roles of individual users as part of an organization (Brickner 2020b, 297).

100. b A consolidated federated model has independent vaults or databases managed by the health information organization (HIO) so that data are centrally managed but both logically and physically separated (Amatayakul 2020, 347–348).

CCA Practice Exam 2

1. c The residual condition or nature of the sequela is sequenced first, followed by the cause of the sequela (Schraffenberger and Palkie 2022, 38–39). The seventh character S is added to the laceration code to identify the sequela.

2. a Per CPT guidelines, when a lesion is excised and the resultant defect is closed with adjacent tissue transfer, only the tissue transfer is coded. See definitions preceding code 14000. Examples of adjacent tissue transfers include Z-plasty, W-plasty, V–Y-plasty, rotation flap, advancement flap, and double-pedicle flap. It is inappropriate to assign an excision code along with an adjacent tissue transfer code (Smith 2021, 79).

3. b Traumatic amputation is classified in Chapter 19. Index Traumatic amputation, finger (complete metacarpophalangeal) S68.11-. seventh character A initial encounter (Schraffenberger and Palkie 2022, 606).

4. c Bypass qualifier specifies the body part bypassed to (Kuehn and Jorwic 2022, 43; CMS 2022a, B3.6a).

5. b Near-syncope and nausea are both symptoms and therefore not integral to the other. Both conditions should be coded (Schraffenberger and Palkie 2022, 565–566).

6. **d** An oral glucose tolerance test helps determine whether a patient has prediabetes or diabetes. Index Elevated, elevation, glucose tolerance (oral) R73.02, which when verified in the Tabular, is a complete code. The Tabular should always be referenced to verify the code (Schraffenberger and Palkie 2022, 202–204).

7. **a** The root operation Extraction D is assigned because a form of instrumentation was used to extract the products of conception. Approach 7 through natural opening is assigned. The qualifier 7 is assigned for the internal version (Kuehn and Jorwic 2022, 414).

8. **a** Code signs and symptoms when a condition is *ruled out,* which means the condition has been proven not to exist. The code for seizures (R56.9) is assigned when a more specific diagnosis cannot be made even after all the facts bearing on the case have been investigated (Schraffenberger and Palkie 2022, 689).

9. **c** Urinary incontinence is a loss of urine without warning and may be associated with many conditions. ICD-10-CM classifies stress incontinence to N39.3 for both male and female types. Index Incontinence, stress (female) (male), N39.3. Subcategory N39.4, Other specified urinary incontinence, provides additional specificity that is not documented in this case.

Code N39.46, Mixed incontinence, is not correct because it includes urge incontinence in addition to stress. The patient only had stress incontinence. Code R32, Unspecified urinary incontinence, is not correct due to Excludes 1 note which excludes N39.3. Code N39.498, Other specified urinary incontinence, is not correct because the type (stress) has a specific code (Schraffenberger and Palkie 2022, 465–466).

10. **c** Assign sepsis for principal as "code first the infection." Index: Sepsis (generalized)(unspecified organism) Category Z16, Resistance to Antimicrobial Drugs, is used as additional code (Schraffenberger and Palkie 2022, 687, 668–670).

11. **a** Parentheses enclose supplementary words or explanatory information that may or may not be present in the statement of a diagnosis or procedure. They do not affect the code number assigned in the case. Bronchiectasis (fusiform) (postinfectious) (recurrent) is an example of a diagnosis statement with nonessential modifiers noted with parentheses (Schraffenberger and Palkie 2022, 23).

12. **a** Each main section of the CPT code manual is divided into subsections, subcategories, headings, and procedures/services (Smith 2021, 18).

13. **a** Per Coding Guideline I.C.13.c, the seventh character A is used as long as the patient is receiving active treatment for the fracture. While the patient may be seen by a new or different provider over the course of treatment for the pathological fracture, assignment of the seventh character is based on whether the patient is undergoing active treatment and not whether the provider is seeing the patient for the first time (CMS 2022a).

14. **c** The terms *metastatic to* and *direct extension to* are used for classifying secondary malignant neoplasms in ICD-10-CM. For example, cancer described as "metastatic to a specific site" is interpreted as a secondary neoplasm of that site. The colon (C18.9) is the primary site, and the left lung (C78.02) is the secondary site (Schraffenberger and Palkie 2022, 145–146).

15. **b** A note appearing after a specific CPT code that instructs the coding professional not to assign that code as a single code. It must be used with another code (Smith 2021, 21, 26).

16. c ICD-10-CM classifies inadequately controlled, out of control, and poorly controlled diabetes mellitus as "*code* to diabetes, by type, with hyperglycemia." In this case, diabetes, diabetic, type 2, with, hyperglycemia. Malnutrition, mild, not stated as related to diabetes Index: Malnutrition, degree, mild E44.1 (Schraffenberger and Palkie 2022, 192–194).

17. c An organ donor match indicates the organ to be transplanted was taken from a different individual of the same species, which is also known as an allogeneic transplant. The Alphabetic Index main term is Transplantation, Kidney, Right 0TY00Z. Reference the 0TY table for the remaining characters of the code. The body part value is the right kidney (0), the approach is open (0), the device is none (0), and the qualifier is allogeneic (0), resulting in code 0TY00Z0 (Kuehn and Jorwic 2022, 97–98).

18. c All the E/M services "roll up into" the most intensive service, which is the hospital admission visit. See definitions preceding code 99201. Individual codes should not be assigned for the visits prior to the admission, although the medical decision-making that occurred then would be a part of the medical decision-making for the hospital admission (Smith 2021, 250; AMA 2021, 19).

19. b New technology is addressed by the Category III codes (Smith 2021, 4).

20. b A procedure may be coded separately when it is not performed as part of another, larger service; and may be reported separately (AMA 2021, 9).

21. c Total abdominal hysterectomy is coded 58150, Total Abdominal Hysterectomy with or without removal of tubes, with or without the removal of ovaries. Modifier 80 identifies the assistant surgeon (Smith 2021, 57).

22. c Any physician may use the codes in any section of CPT (Smith 2021, 30–31).

23. d See instructional notes preceding code 99217. In order to report these codes, the admission order must designate observation status. Whether the patient meets admission criteria or is admitted following surgery does not affect the observation code selection. If the patient is admitted and discharged on the same date, codes 99234–99236 are appropriate (AMA 2021, 21).

24. b Documentation of history of use of drugs, alcohol, and tobacco is part of the social history. The review of systems is a part of the history of present illness. See E/M Services Guidelines, instructions for selecting a level of E/M service, in the CPT manual (AMA 2021, 10).

25. c Tissue transplanted from one individual to another of the same species but different genotype is called an allograft or allogeneic graft (Smith 2021, 90).

26. a The "with manipulation" code is used because the fracture was manipulated, even if the manipulation did not result in clinical anatomic alignment. See Musculoskeletal Guidelines, Definitions (AMA 2021, 139–140).

27. d Newborn care services are used to report the services provided to newborns in several different settings. For the newborn admitted and discharged on the same day, E/M code assignment per day is 99463 (AMA 2021, 56).

28. a If the tip of the catheter is manipulated, it is a selective catheterization. In the case of a nonselective catheterization, the tip of the catheter remains in either the aorta or the artery that was originally entered (Smith 2021, 130).

29. **b** Attending and consulting physicians have no bearing on the assignment of the MS-DRG and payment to the hospital (Schraffenberger and Palkie 2022, 724–726).

30. **a** All the statements are true except this one. The Category III codes are updated every six months in order to reflect current advances in technology (Smith 2021, 24).

31. **a** For S82.251A, the Alphabetic Index main term is Fracture, traumatic, subterms tibia (shaft), comminuted (displaced) S82.25-. The Tabular List is consulted to assign the sixth character 1 for displaced right and seventh character A for initial encounter for closed fracture. A fracture not indicated as open or closed is coded closed and a fracture not indicated as displaced or not displaced is coded to displaced (CMS 2022a, I.C.19.c). For S06.0X0A, the Alphabetic Index main term is Concussion, without loss of consciousness (S06.0X0). The Tabular List is reviewed to assign sixth character 0 representing without loss of consciousness and seventh character A for initial encounter. For S50.359A the Alphabetic Index main term is Splinter, see Foreign body, superficial, by site; superficial, without open wound, elbow S50.35-. For W01.198A, the External Cause Alphabetic Index main term is Fall, subterm due to, slipping, with subsequent striking against object, specified NEC. The Tabular List is consulted to assign seventh character A for initial encounter. For Y92.480, the Alphabetic Index main term is Place of occurrence, subterm street or highway, sidewalk. For Y93.K1, the External Cause Alphabetic Index main term is Activity, subterm walking an animal. For Y99.8, the External Cause Alphabetic Index main term is External cause status, subterm specified NEC. Code Y92.480, Y93.K1 and Y99.8 are POA exempt. The other conditions were present on admission. The Alphabetic Index main term is Reposition, subterms tibia, right. Table 0QS is reviewed to assign approach value 0 for open and device value 4 for internal fixation device (CMS 2022b, 2.6).

32. **b** Diagnosis codes are often the primary reason for a service to be considered covered or denied by the insurance company. Local and national policies include diagnosis codes that are used in software edits to automatically deny or approve processed claims. Denied services can be appealed, and the record can be submitted to support medical necessity if the service fails the automated review (Schraffenberger and Palkie 2022, 723–724).

33. **b** The National Uniform Billing Committee (NUBC) was established with the goal of developing an acceptable, uniform bill that would consolidate the numerous billing forms hospitals were required to use (Smith 2021, 15).

34. **a** OPPS requires that facilities use HCPCS code to report services or procedures performed. Each code in HCPCS has been assigned a payment status indicator (SI) that establishes how a service, procedure, or item is paid (Casto and White 2021, 105–117).

35. **a** For fiscal year 2008, Medicare adopted a severity-adjusted diagnosis-related groups system called Medicare Severity-DRGs (MS-DRGs). This was the most drastic revision to the DRG system in 24 years. The goal of the MS-DRG system was to significantly improve Medicare's ability to recognize severity of illness in its inpatient hospital payments. The new system is projected to increase payments to hospitals for services provided to the sicker patients and decrease payments for treating less severely ill patients (Schraffenberger and Palkie 2022, 724–726).

36. **a** For any given patient in a MS-DRG, the hospital knows, in advance, the amount of reimbursement it will receive from Medicare. It is the responsibility of the hospital to ensure that its resource use is in line with the payment (Casto and White 2021, 210–211).

37. d Medicare provides for additional payment for other factors related to a particular hospital's business. If the hospital treats a high percentage of low-income patients, it receives a percentage add-on payment applied to the MS-DRG adjusted base payment rate. This add-on payment, known as the disproportionate share hospital (DSH) adjustment, provides for a percentage increase in Medicare payments to hospitals that qualify under either of two statutory formulas designed to identify hospitals that serve these areas. Hospitals that have approved teaching hospitals also receive a percentage add-on payment for each Medicare discharge paid under IPPS, known as the indirect medical education (IME) adjustment. The percentage varies, depending on the ratio of residents to beds. Additional payments are made for new technologies or medical services that have been approved for special add-on payments. Finally, the costs incurred by a hospital for a Medicare beneficiary are evaluated to determine whether the hospital is eligible for an additional payment as an outlier case. This additional payment is designed to protect the hospital from large financial losses due to unusually expensive cases (Schraffenberger and Palkie 2022, 727).

38. b Congress directed HHS to conduct a three-year demonstration project using recovery audit contractors (RACs) to detect and correct improper payments in the Medicare traditional fee-for-service program. Congress further required HHS to make the RAC program permanent and nationwide by January 1, 2010 (Schraffenberger and Palkie 2022, 734–735).

39. a ICD-10-CM diagnosis codes are the foundation of the CMS Hierarchical Condition Categories (HCCs), as they directly impact the risk score calculation (Casto and White 2021, 60).

40. d The chargemaster, or charge description master (CDM), is a database used by healthcare facilities to house billing information for all services provided to patients (Casto and White 2021, 144–153).

41. b Billing for two services that are prohibited from being billed on the same day would be identified by the NCCI edits (Smith 2021, 69–70).

42. c Remittance advice (RA) is sent to the provider to explain payments made by third-party payers (Casto and White 2021, 168).

43. b The monies collected from third-party payers cannot be greater than the amount of the provider's charges (Casto and White 2021, 51–58).

44. c The purpose of a physician query is to improve documentation to support services billed (Brinda 2020, 186).

45. c To qualify for a cost outlier, a hospital's charges for a case (adjusted to cost) must exceed the payment rate for the MS-DRG by a specific threshold amount determined by CMS for each fiscal year (Casto and White 2021, 74, 80).

46. c The Medicare National Coverage Determinations (NCD) Manual is an internet-only manual (IOM) published by CMS that provides a listing of all topics included in active NCDs (Casto and White 2021, 215).

47. a Developed by third-party payers, a fee schedule is a list of healthcare services and procedures and the charges associated with each (Casto and White 2021, 52–53).

48. b   The charge description master includes the charge code; charge code description; CPT/HCPCS code and modifier; revenue code; and price. It does not contain the MS-DRG assignment (Casto and White 2021, 144–153).

49. a   An advance beneficiary notice (ABN) must be given to the patient to sign before treatment if any indication presents that may cause the service to be denied by Medicare (Casto and White 2021, 137–139).

50. a   When a physician accepts assignment of benefits, the physician can only collect any applicable deductible or coinsurance from the patient (Casto and White 2021, 125, 243).

51. c   Budget neutrality must be maintained annually when the relative value units (RVUs) are adjusted (Hazelwood 2020, 232–234).

52. b   The status indicator (SI) N identifies procedures, services, and supplies that are packaged into the cost and reimbursement for APC services with which they are most often performed (Casto and White 2021, 113).

53. d   Only confirmed cases of HIV infection or illness are reported, using code B20, Human immunodeficiency virus (HIV) disease, per ICD-10-CM Official Guidelines for Coding and Reporting, Guideline I.C.1.a.1 (CMS 2022a).

       Patients with an HIV-related illness should be coded to category B20, which includes AIDS, AIDS-like syndrome, AIDS-related complex, and symptomatic HIV infection. B20, Human immunodeficiency virus, is the first-listed diagnosis code when a patient is seen for an HIV-related condition. Any HIV-related conditions should be listed as additional diagnosis codes (Schraffenberger and Palkie 2022, 130–133).

54. b   The connecting term "due to" connects the organism *E. coli* to the urinary tract infection. The instructional note "Use additional code" (B95–B97) is found in the Tabular List of ICD-10-CM under Code N39.0. This notation indicates that use of an additional code may provide a more complete picture of the diagnosis or procedure. The additional code should always be assigned if the health record provides supportive documentation. Infection, urinary (tract) Tabular List—use additional code to identify organism. Infection, *Escherichia coli*. Index: Infection, Escherichia (E.) coli NEC, as cause of disease classified elsewhere B96.20 (Schraffenberger and Palkie 2022, 33–34).

55. a   The name of surgeon and assistants, date, duration, and description of the procedure and any specimens removed are found in the operative report (Brickner 2020a, 108–109).

56. a   Present on admission is defined as present at the time the order for inpatient admission occurs (CMS 2022c, Appendix I).

57. b   Medical history documents the patient's current complaints and symptoms and lists the patient's past medical, personal, and family history. The physical examination report represents the attending physician's assessment of the patient's current health status (Smith 2021, 223–247).

58. d   The goal of documentation standards is to ensure the content of the health record so that it can be used for patient care (Brickner 2020a, 95–100).

59. a   All patients meeting the United Network of Organ Sharing (UNOS) criteria must be evaluated with the documentation part of the health record per CMS and the Joint Commission (Sharp 2020, 208).

60. **b** A consultation report records the opinion of any physician who is asked by the patient's physician to provide advice on the patient's care (Brickner 2020a, 104).

61. **c** The American College of Surgeons started its Hospital Standardization Program in 1918 (Sharp 2020, 204).

62. **c** All entries must be legible and complete and must be authenticated and dated promptly by the person (identified by name and discipline) who is responsible for ordering, providing, or evaluating the service furnished (42 CFR 482.24).

63. **d** In a paper-based health record environment, when corrections are made to health record entries, it is appropriate to draw a single line through the original entry, write "error" above the entry, and then sign the correction, including the date and time (Sayles 2020, 78, 83, 139).

64. **a** Qualitative analysis is about the quality of the documentation including the use of approved abbreviations (Sayles 2020, 76).

65. **b** External clinical validation audits are typically conducted on Medicare patients' health records by the Recovery Audit Contractor (RAC) (Foltz and Lankisch 2020, 515).

66. **a** The physician principally responsible for the patient's hospital care writes and signs the discharge summary (Brickner 2020a, 109).

67. **a** Histology refers to the tissue type of a lesion. The histology of tissue is determined by a pathologist and documented in the pathology report (Schraffenberger and Palkie 2022, 153).

68. **a** The problem list describes any significant current and past illnesses and conditions as well as the procedures the patient has undergone (Amatayakul 2020, 334).

69. **b** Data quality needs to be consistent. A difference in the use of abbreviations provides a good example of how the lack of consistency can lead to problems (Brickner 2020b, 295).

70. **d** Access control means being able to identify which employees should have access to what data (Brickner 2020b, 297–298, 311).

71. **a** HIM ethical obligations apply regardless of employment site (Hamilton 2020, 671–674).

72. **a** Corrective action should be taken when error or accuracy rates are deemed to be at an unacceptable rate (Sayles 2020, 76).

73. **d** Standards are fixed rules that must be followed, and vary from guidelines that provide general direction (Sayles 2020, 79, 95–96).

74. **c** Healthcare organizations should have a coding compliance plan in addition to the organization's compliance plan, with the same components (Rinehart-Thompson 2020b, 279).

75. **d** The addendum must have a separate signature, date, and time from the original entry (Sayles 2020, 88).

76. **a** The Joint Commission, Commission on Accreditation of Rehabilitation Facilities, and the National Committee for Quality Assurance are all acceptable accrediting bodies for behavioral healthcare settings (Brickner 2020a, 97, 99–100).

77. **c** State licensure agencies have regulations that are modeled after the Medicare Conditions of Participation and Joint Commission standards. States conduct annual surveys to determine the hospital's continued compliance with licensure standards (Rinehart-Thompson 2020b, 248–249).

78. **a** The CDM captures charges for services including accommodations, room use, supplies, ancillary provisions and clinical services (Gordon 2020, 476).

79. **d** The pre-claims submission activities include tasks and functions that can accurately establish the patient's financial class (Casto and White 2022, 234).

80. **c** A goal of the CDI program is to identify and clarify missing, conflicting or non-specific physician documentation related to diagnoses and procedures (Brinda 2020, 188).

81. **c** An addendum may be included in the health record to update or supplement documentation that has been recorded (Sayles 2020, 78, 81, 102).

82. **d** Recovery audit contractors (RACs) work to reduce Medicare improper payments through detection and collection of overpayments, the identification of underpayments, and the implementation of actions that will prevent future improper payments (Casto and White 2021, 204–207).

83. **c** Edit checks help ensure data integrity by allowing only reasonable and predetermined values to be entered into the computer (Brickner 2020b, 301).

84. **b** When several people enter data in an EHR, you can define how users must enter data in specific fields to help maintain consistency. For example, an input mask for a form means that users can only enter the date in a specified format (Sayles 2020, 83).

85. **b** CAC can help prevent fraudulent coding and ensure complete, consistent coding due to the NLP (Foltz and Lankisch 2020, 520).

86. **a** An encoder is computer software that helps the coding professional assign codes (Sayles 2020, 87).

87. **c** Natural language processing (NLP) uses artificial intelligence software to allow digital text from online documents stored in the organization's information system to be read directly by the software, which then suggests codes to match the documentation (Sayles 2020, 82, 331, 368).

88. **b** Each time the patient visits the facility, the same health record number is used, allowing communication between past and present healthcare providers and consistent sharing of information regarding the course of treatment (Sayles 2020, 73–80).

89. **c** Computer-assisted coding utilizes computer software to generate codes from the data provided (Sayles 2020, 83).

90. **b** The foundation of CAC that converts the human words into data that can be translated and manipulated by the computer system is natural language processing (Casto and White 2021, 183).

91. **b** People are the greatest threat to electronic health information (Brickner 2020b, 288).

92. c   Section 4004 of the 21st Century Cures Act identifies eight exceptions that offer actors (healthcare providers, health IT developers, HINs, and HIEs) certainty that when their practices access, exchange, or use health information that meet those conditions, the practice will not be considered information blocking (HealthIT.gov 2022).

93. b   An EHR can be viewed by multiple users and from multiple locations at any time, and organizations must have in place appropriate security access control measures to ensure the safety of the data (Sayles 2020, 80–87).

94. a   The method of encryption when two or more computers share the same secret key which is used to both encrypt and decrypt a message is called private key infrastructure or single-key encryption (Brickner 2020b, 302).

95. a   Privacy is the right of an individual to be left alone (Rinehart-Thompson 2020b, 248).

96. b   HIPAA states that state law preempts the HIPAA Privacy Rule (Rinehart-Thompson 2020b, 249).

97. d   Confidentiality is the area responsible for limiting disclosure (Rinehart-Thompson 2020b, 248).

98. b   A blanket authorization is a common ethical problem when misused. Patients often sign a blanket authorization, which authorizes the release of information from that point forward, without understanding the implications. The problem is the patient is not aware of what information is being accessed (Hamilton 2020, 671).

99. d   A covered entity may either account for the disclosures of its business associate or require the business associate to make their own accounting. The business associate must respond to accounting requests made directly to them (Rinehart-Thompson 2020b, 257).

100. a   States license hospitals in order to treat patients. Further regulations include record maintenance and continuing education (Rinehart-Thompson 2020a, 240).

REFERENCES

42 CFR 482.24: Medical Record Services. 2022.

Amatayakul, M. K. 2020. Health Information Technologies. Chapter 11 in *Health Information Management Technology: An Applied Approach*, 6th ed. Edited by N. B. Sayles and L. L. Gordon. Chicago: AHIMA.

American Health Information Management Association. 2020. *Clinical Coding Workout: Practice Exercises for Skill Development with Answers*, 2020 ed. Chicago: AHIMA.

American Medical Association. 2021. *CPT Current Procedural Terminology Professional Edition*. Chicago: AMA.

Bowe, H. and L. M. Williamson. 2020. Healthcare Information. Chapter 12 in *Health Information Management Technology: An Applied Approach*, 6th ed. Edited by N. B. Sayles and L. L. Gordon. Chicago: AHIMA.

Brickner, M. R. 2020a. Health Record Content and Documentation. Chapter 4 in *Health Information Management Technology: An Applied Approach*, 6th ed. Edited by N. B. Sayles and L. L. Gordon. Chicago: AHIMA.

Brickner, M. R. 2020b. Data Security. Chapter 10 in *Health Information Management Technology: An Applied Approach*, 6th ed. Edited by N. B. Sayles and L. L. Gordon. Chicago: AHIMA.

Brinda, D. 2020. Data Management. Chapter 6 in *Health Information Management Technology: An Applied Approach*, 6th ed. Edited by N. B. Sayles and L. L. Gordon. Chicago: AHIMA.

Brinda, D. and A. Watters. 2020. Data Privacy, Confidentiality, and Security. Chapter 11 in *Health Information Management: Concepts, Principles, and Practice*, 6th ed. Edited by P. Oachs and A. Watters. Chicago: AHIMA.

Casto, A. and S. White. 2021. *Principles of Healthcare Reimbursement and Revenue Cycle Management*, 7th ed. Chicago: AHIMA.

Centers for Medicare and Medicaid Services (CMS). 2022a. ICD-10-CM Official Guidelines for Coding and Reporting. https://www.cms.gov/files/document/fy-2022-icd-10-cm-coding-guidelines -updated-02012022.pdf.

Centers for Medicare and Medicaid Services (CMS). 2022b. National Correct Coding Initiative Policy Manual for Medicare Services. https://www.cms.gov/files/document /chapter1generalcorrectcodingpoliciesfinal11.pdf.

Centers for Medicare and Medicaid Services (CMS). 2022c. ICD-10-PCS Reference Manual. https://www.cms.gov/files/document/2022-official-icd-10-pcs-coding-guidelines-updated -december-1-2021.pdf.

Foltz, D. A. and K. M. Lankisch. 2020. Fraud and Abuse Compliance. Chapter 16 in *Health Information Management Technology: An Applied Approach*, 6th ed. Edited by N. B. Sayles and L. L. Gordon. Chicago: AHIMA.

Giannangelo, K. 2019. *Healthcare Code Sets, Clinical Terminologies, and Classification Systems*. Chicago: AHIMA.

Gordon, M. L. 2020. Revenue Management and Reimbursement. Chapter 15 in *Health Information Management Technology: An Applied Approach*, 6th ed. Edited by N. B. Sayles and L. L. Gordon. Chicago: AHIMA.

Hamilton, M. 2020. Ethical Issues in Health Information Management. Chapter 21 in *Health Information Management Technology: An Applied Approach*, 6th ed. Edited by N. B. Sayles and L. L. Gordon. Chicago: AHIMA.

Handlon, L. 2020. Revenue Cycle Management. Chapter 8 in *Health Information Management: Concepts, Principles, and Practice*, 6th ed. Edited by P. Oachs and A. Watters. Chicago: AHIMA.

Hazelwood, A. C. and C. A. Venable. 2020. Reimbursement Methodologies. Chapter 7 in *Health Information Management: Concepts, Principles, and Practice*, 6th ed. Edited by P. Oachs and A. Watters. Chicago: AHIMA.

HealthIT.gov. 2022. ONC's Cures Act Final Rule. https://www.healthit.gov/curesrule/.

Hunt, T. J. and K. Kirk. 2020. Clinical Documentation Integrity and Coding Compliance. Chapter 9 in *Health Information Management: Concepts, Principles, and Practice*, 6th ed. Edited by P. Oachs and A. Watters. Chicago: AHIMA.

Johns, M. 2020. Governing Data and Information Assets. Chapter 3 in *Health Information Management: Concepts, Principles, and Practice*, 6th ed. Edited by P. Oachs and A. Watters. Chicago: AHIMA.

Kuehn, L. and T. Jorwic. 2021. *ICD-10-PCS: An Applied Approach*. Chicago: AHIMA.

LeBlanc, M. 2020. Human Resources Management and Professional Development. Chapter 20 in *Health Information Management Technology: An Applied Approach*, 6th ed. Edited by N. B. Sayles and L. L. Gordon. Chicago: AHIMA.

Miller, K. 2020. Healthcare Delivery Systems. Chapter 2 in *Health Information Management Technology: An Applied Approach*, 6th ed. Edited by N. B. Sayles and L. L. Gordon. Chicago: AHIMA.

O'Dell, R. M. 2020. Clinical Quality Management. Chapter 20 in *Health Information Management: Concepts, Principles, and Practice*, 6th ed. Edited by P. Oachs and A. Watters. Chicago: AHIMA.

Palkie, B. 2020. Clinical Classifications, Vocabularies, Terminologies, and Standards. Chapter 5 in *Health Information Management: Concepts, Principles, and Practice*, 6th ed. Edited by P. Oachs and A. Watters. Chicago: AHIMA.

Primeau, D., J. Pursley, and L. Riplinger. 2021 (February 10). Five Strategies for Your Organization's Information Blocking Plan. https://journal.ahima.org/five-strategies-for-your-organizations-information-blocking-plan/.

Prater, V. S. 2020. Human Resources Management. Chapter 20 in *Health Information Management Technology: An Applied Approach*, 6th ed. Edited by N. B. Sayles and L. L. Gordon. Chicago: AHIMA.

Reynolds, R. B. and A. Morey. 2020. Health Record Content and Documentation. Chapter 4 in *Health Information Management: Concepts, Principles, and Practice*, 6th ed. Edited by P. Oachs and A. Watters. Chicago: AHIMA.

Rinehart-Thompson, L. A. 2020a. Health Law. Chapter 8 in *Health Information Management Technology: An Applied Approach*, 6th ed. Edited by N. B. Sayles and L. L. Gordon. Chicago: AHIMA.

Rinehart-Thompson, L. A. 2020b. Data Privacy and Confidentiality. Chapter 9 in *Health Information Management Technology: An Applied Approach*, 6th ed. Edited by N. B. Sayles and L. L. Gordon. Chicago: AHIMA.

Sayles, N. B. 2020. Health Information Functions, Purpose, and Users. Chapter 3 in *Health Information Management Technology: An Applied Approach*, 6th ed. Edited by N. B. Sayles and L. L. Gordon. Chicago: AHIMA.

Sayles, N. B. and L. L. Gordon, eds. 2020. *Health Information Management Technology: An Applied Approach*, 6th ed. Chicago: AHIMA.

Schraffenberger, L. A. and Palkie, B. 2022. *Basic ICD-10-CM and ICD-10-PCS Coding*. Chicago: AHIMA.

Scott, K. 2020. *Coding and Reimbursement for Hospital Inpatient Services*, 4th ed. Chicago: AHIMA.

Sharp, M. Y. 2020. Secondary Data Sources. Chapter 7 in *Health Information Management Technology: An Applied Approach*, 6th ed. Edited by N. B. Sayles and L. L. Gordon. Chicago: AHIMA.

Smith, G. 2021. *Basic Current Procedural Terminology and HCPCS Coding*. Chicago: AHIMA.

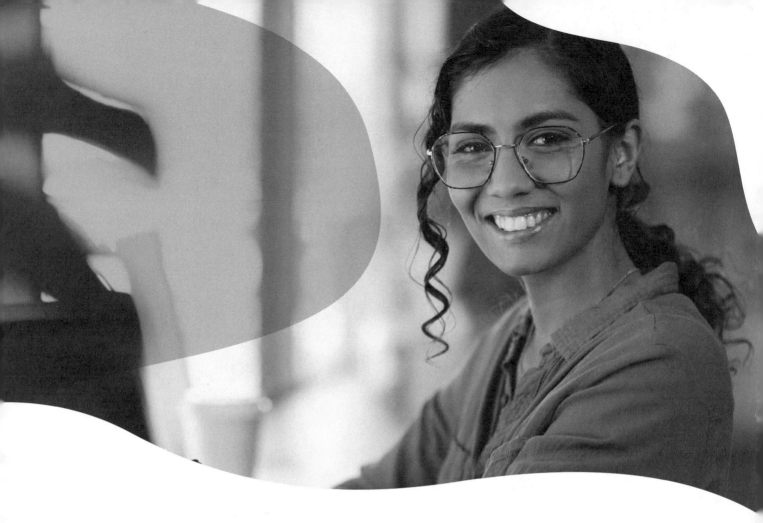

Discover, Connect, Advance

Join AHIMA, and join a community of passionate, forward-thinking health information professionals driving progress in the world of healthcare.

As an AHIMA student member, you will enjoy a variety of benefits:

- Discounts in the AHIMA Store on resources, like textbooks and certification exam prep
- Support for your schoolwork through AHIMA's HIM Body of Knowledge™
- AHIMA Foundation scholarships eligibility
- Timely articles weekly through the Journal of AHIMA and the E-alert email newsletter
- Career coaches, resume reviewers, and early access to new jobs posted on the Career Assist: Job Bank
- Networking opportunities at the state and national level
- The members-only social platform Access, where you can discuss the latest AHIMA articles and hot topics, talk with and learn from other members, and explore and share AHIMA education and news
- Empowerment to participate in advocacy and public policy through our Take Action Center

Join today at ahima.org/join

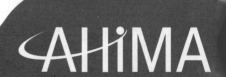